Autoimmune Protocol Diet

The Complete Guide to the Protocol to Improving Your Health With the Autoimmune Diet

Alexander Great

any responsibility of actions taken by the reader in conjunction with this work. The Publisher acknowledges that the reader acts of their own accord and releases the author and Publisher of any responsibility for the observance of tips, advice, counsel, strategies, and techniques that may be offered in this volume.

Tablet of Contents

Introduction

Chapter 2: Autoimmune Diseases and What they Are.

Introduction

Congratulations on purchasing *Autoimmune Protocol Diet,* and thank you for also choosing this book. Throughout the following pages, I hope you find the answers to the many questions you might have regarding eating for autoimmune issues. The Autoimmune Diet Protocol or *AIP* is a relatively recent popular diet in the marketplace, and there are many questions concerning eating the right anti-inflammatory foods to maintain a healthy gut and immune system.

So, what is an autoimmune disease? An autoimmune disease is a disorder whereby the immune system begins to attack healthy cells. The body then dives into overdrive in response, causing inflammation in various parts of the body. The result is a significant disruption of regular bodily functions. This disruption causes considerable change to lifestyle and dietary changes. Until recently, compared to other popular diet movements, little attention in the popular marketplace was paid to autoimmune diets. However, as we better understand our immune systems, improved diet dietary advice, and diet protocols have come along, offering a higher level of understanding and control over our dietary choices.

Within the pages of this book, in addition to understanding the Autoimmune Diet Protocol, we will look at some of the reasons our immune system may *attack* itself, causing flare-ups. We will also look at the elimination of certain foods in our diet, in addition to talking about good and bad fats, and the positive role supplements may play in supporting our healthy dietary and immunity-boosting choices.

We hope you enjoy reading this book and gain a significant lifestyle and nutritional improvement from it.

Thanks again for choosing this book, make sure to leave a short review on Amazon if you enjoy it, I'd really love to hear your thoughts.

Get the audiobook version of this title for free with a 30-day Audible trial

Click here if you are from the US:
https://www.audible.com/pd/B08GNGVXW8/?source_code=AUDFPWS0223189MWT-BK-ACX0-213727&ref=acx_bty_BK_ACX0_213727_rh_us

Click here if you are from the UK:
https://www.audible.co.uk/pd/B08GN4Y35X/?source_code=AUKFrDlWS0223189OH6-BK-ACX0-213727&ref=acx_bty_BK_ACX0_213727_rh_uk

Click here if you are from the FR:
https://www.audible.fr/pd/B08GNFLPKN/?source_code=FRAORWS022318903B-BK-ACX0-213727&ref=acx_bty_BK_ACX0_213727_rh_fr

Click here if you are from the DE:
https://www.audible.de/pd/B08GND242L/?source_code=EKAORWS0223189009-BK-ACX0-213727&ref=acx_bty_BK_ACX0_213727_rh_de

Chapter 1: The Autoimmune Diet Protocol

The Autoimmune Diet Protocol (AIP) is pretty new to the marketplace. It is essentially a food-based method of minimizing inflammatory responses or eliminating unwelcome inflammation. The inflammation over the intestine caused by various conditions may be improved by the removal of certain foods like nuts and beans from a person's diet.

The Auto-Immune Diet Protocol. More than another Fad

The diet is restrictive. Therefore, for somebody who is otherwise healthy and only looking for a better way to eat, this diet may take some discipline.

For somebody, however, dealing with the very real consequences and lifestyle encroachments caused by an autoimmune inflammatory disease, following a diet specifically tailored to the issue may feel liberating. Once the foods that are considered provocative are ruled out, then it may be possible to resume a healthy lifestyle.

Essentially, the idea behind the Autoimmune Diet Protocol is to reduce the inflammation within your body. For those dealing with autoimmune conditions, it may be possible to go into remission through better food choices, resulting in a better quality of life.

You might also have heard about Leaky Gut, as something associated with an autoimmune condition. Leaky gut refers to the presence of small holes within the intestines caused or certainly aggravated by gassy producing foods such as high protein beans and some vegetables. Following the restrictive protocol of this diet provides an opportunity to heal the gut, hopefully producing a positive outcome for overall health and wellness.

Going through this book, you might think this diet is very much like the Paleo Diet. So why not just follow the Paleo Diet?

The Paleo Diet, while being restrictive, still permits some of the food choices not allowed on the Autoimmune Diet Protocol. For example, the Paleo Diet allows the consumption of eggs and nuts. The AIP diet does not.

The AIP diet also asks dieters to avoid painkillers like ibuprofen and aspirin and naproxen. If you are taking any of these medications as part of a treatment or pain management program, you might want to consult a health care professional for alternative remedies during this diet program.

Leaky Gut, Blood Sugar, and the Importance of Supporting our Immune System.

In any medical situation, the key to understanding underlying symptoms is crucial. The Autoimmune Diet attempts to improve inflammatory symptoms, returning wellness to the immune system, balancing it once more.

1. Gut health: Gut Inflammation, Gut Dysbiosis (imbalances in gut bacteria), and a leaky lining of the gut cause a restriction of nutrient absorption, resulting in inflammation; these issues harm the autoimmune reaction. The purpose of the diet is to correct these issues and prevent further damage.

2. Density: So, our body may function at its maximum potential; it requires a variety of nutrients to function at its best. Foods, of course, are vital in the production of resources moving throughout the body. It is these resources that maximize healing under stress, therefore supporting the immune system

3. Blood Sugar: Both low and high blood sugar have the potential to cause inflammation and hormonal imbalance. Without this, even brain function becomes compromised. Supporting healthy blood flow, balanced glucose levels are crucial for the rebalancing of inflammatory conditions. This diet may provide long term solutions that are essential in promoting blood to sugar balance.

4. System regulation: Leaky Gut, Inflammation, Blood Sugar Imbalances, Hormone Imbalances, can all be better supported and possibly healed from further damage through inflammation by eating

according to an improved immune response diet such as the Autoimmune Diet Protocol.

Immunity, Guts, and the Brain Connection

Did you know that the gut and the brain, regarding mood issues such as depression and anxiety, are entirely connected? The health of our gut may be an indicator of the health of our minds! Equally, our mental state can affect gut health through anxiety and stress. This may explain why medical professionals propose a diet rich in fresh, organic produce as essential for those dealing with mental health issues.
This marriage between the brain and the gut also applies to unpredictable mood patterns. Problems with wildly fluctuating mood are now known to be associated with gastrointestinal symptoms. Worth noting, mood swings are now known for their link to functional digestive disorders such as Irritable Bowel Syndrome.

Problems with the gut may be implicated in the diagnosis of mood disorders when individuals dealing with sudden and unpredictable mood swings present abnormal physical symptoms. Crohn's Disease patients, for example, may have a higher than the normal number of high and low dips in emotional swings. Surgical patients reported lower levels of mood elevations, peaks, and troughs. Something that might be expected when dealing with an undercurrent of neurological issues.

So, why do gut problems cause mood swings and other mental health problems? Well, the gut is a significant producer of serotonin, the neurotransmitter that regulates our moods. Additionally, changes in healthy gut flora have the potential to affect both mental health, and of course, attitude.

Anyone dealing with unpredictable levels of emotional responses and intestinal related matters stemming from autoimmune issues to include Irritable Bowel Syndrome, the two points may be connected. To complicate things even more, not all problems with the gut, present inflammatory symptoms in the abdomen!

Notorious for this is Celiac Disease: often, primary symptoms that present are epidermal irritations on the surface of the skin, or mental health problems, as opposed to an upset stomach or the abdominal pain one might think.

When we think about the brain and the gut connection, a diet targeted to healing and even arresting further gut damage is an attractive lifestyle choice.

Paleo Versus Paleo AIP. How Does This Diet Compare?

The Paleo Autoimmune Protocol or AIP is essentially the Paleo diet but with a more significant number of limitations. The aim of the Paleo AIP is the eradication of any type of food with a history of kicking the immune system into overdrive. These restrictions are in addition to dairy, corn, soy, and processed foods. Other foods have demonstrated a trend for causing problems being in people with Inflammatory Diseases.

On either diet, the primary method of investigating problematic foods, and understanding the ones that are not, is to cut all of them from your diet. After approximately sixty days, reintroduce them to see how or if you react.

 These food items are allowed on the Paleo diet, marking the slight difference between the two diet protocols.

- dairy to include eggs
- potatoes
- tomatoes
- peppers
- chilis
- eggplant
- seeds
- nuts
- dairy
- clarified butter
- chocolate
- caffeine
- alcohol
- coriander
- fennel
- cardamom

- paprika
- chili powders

GAPS Diet. What It Is

Perhaps you might have heard of the Gut and Psychology Syndrome or GAPS Diet. A similar diet intended to revive the flora in our gut, thus strengthening a weakened immunity. Because of the gut and brain connection, it is believed, among other things, to help individuals dealing with learning disabilities.

The diet places importance on the following variety of nutrient-rich foods:

- Consuming fermented foods
- Supplementing with Probiotics
- Consuming foods rich in vital nutrients, such as dark green leafy vegetables.

Foods best avoided.
- Complex carbohydrates (such as brown rice)
- Wheat gluten and grains
- All sugars, even the natural variation found in honey and maple syrup
- Majority of the nut family
- Majority of beans
- All foods that are processed
- Chemical food additives

- Dairy,
- Alcoholic beverages,
- All fruit juices,
- Caffeinated drinks
- Soda

Besides helping with managing learning disabilities, the GAPS diet has shown improvements in Autoimmune Diseases to include arthritic conditions, anemic disorders, allergic responses such as hay fever, and even the common cold.

Are you preparing for your Autoimmune Diet Protocol? Consider taking these Steps Beforehand.

Before embarking on your Autoimmune Diet Protocol, think about cleaning up your current diet first. During this time, it will prepare you for the more restrictive diet you are about to embark on and may go a long way towards healing some of the inflammation you are currently dealing with.

If you feel better at the start of the diet, it may be an incentive to continue with a more restrictive version for maximum benefit. Remember, this diet involves calorie restriction, one of the side effects of which can be a slower metabolism. The diet is intended to heal your digestive system. The purpose is also to investigate the foods that may be causing sensitivity within your immune system, triggering attacks such as Irritable Bowel Syndrome, and so on.

If you are currently seeking medical advice related to your Autoimmune Diseases, it only makes sense to continue to do so during this time and to speak with your doctor beforehand so that they are aware of the changes you are creating within your diet.

For those of us who are seeking to feel better generally and to improve our overall health, it might be helpful to understand that we are effectively removing a lot of the junk food from our diet. As a result, we may find ourselves craving sugar and even alcohol as we remove toxins from our body!

How to de-tox your current diet:

- Remove *all* foods with sugar as an added ingredient, if you have done this already, great! If not, now is the time to check the labels of everything you will be easting. Hidden sugars are everywhere.

- Remove *all* processed foods. In other words, anything that has more than two ingredients. Specifically, ingredients that you cannot pronounce. Ideally, you should be able to pronounce what is on your food.

- Dispose of inflammatory oils and fats such as Canola based oils. Even the supposed healthy versions of dairy-free snacks and protein bars sometimes contain these fats. Again, this is a time to become label conscious.

- Cease the consumption of artificial sweeteners. Some of these contain the same chlorine chemical compounds found in swimming pools! If that does not put you off, then nothing will!

- Avoid soft drinks, soda, and chemical infused energy drinks. Swap for herbal tea concoctions, or good quality black teas.

- Avoid typical table sauces such as ketchup and dressings for salads and other foods that typically contain sugars or artificial sweeteners.

- Add in some version of fermented food several times a week. Kefir and Kampuchea are readily available at supermarkets for a reasonable price.

- Stop eating out for at least two months before the diet. Make all your meals. If nothing else, your bank account will thank you!

Who should consider using the AIP Diet?

In the next chapter, we will look at specific Autoimmune Diseases; however, the summary below may help you decide if this type of calorie and food choice restrictive diet is right for you.

• Anybody managing one or several related Autoimmune Diseases such as Rheumatoid Arthritis, Multiple Sclerosis, and other similar immune-related diseases.

• Individuals who are managing life-altering and life compromising symptoms that are severe enough to require supportive measures such as physical therapy or modifications throughout the home.

• Anyone whose intolerance or sensitivity to certain food products or ingredients results in a medical or neurological reaction to include depression, anxiety, or a medical emergency.

The common denominator is that patients who have made multiple attempts at diet and lifestyle modifications may want to consider using the Autoimmune Diet Protocol.

Chapter 2: Autoimmune Diseases and What they Are.

The idea of having an immune system that is working too hard is generally not considered to be a bad thing. After all, who does not want to fight off colds, flu, and other viruses? However, the immune system can become overactive. Triggered by stress, mental health issues, and even illness, all of which can cause disruptions in our immune system. This disruption leaves our bodies in a constant state of infection-fighting and inflammatory responses.

What Are Diseases of the Immune System?

In a normally functioning immune system, the body can identify things such as viruses and other pathogens that it does not recognize, before taking necessary measures to destroy these invaders.

However, when issues arise, the immune system begins to attack and destroy its healthy cells. Moreover, these unhealthy, malfunctioning cells hang around, affecting the remaining healthy cells around them. The result is a body that feels under attack and generally run down. When our gut becomes inflamed, as discussed in the previous chapter, we may run the gamut of mood swings to Irritable Bowel Syndrome and a host of other autoimmune response diseases.

What Causes This Type of Disease?

The short answer is that there is no universally agreed upon reason why autoimmune diseases occur. While some types of autoimmune diseases are known for their correlation with variables such as gender, race, and heredity, any exact cause remains unknown.

Some scientists hypothesize that an overactive immune system is caused by food items found in a Western diet, such as excessive fat and sugar. These ingredients can cause inflammation in the body, leading some scientists to believe it is these food additives that trigger an abnormal immune response.

Others, however, attribute overactive immune systems and the resulting autoimmune diseases to the vaccination of children, and the use of antiseptic agents.

Because of modern hygiene practices, immune systems are not exposed to enough germs and pathogens early in life, resulting in excessive immune responses to harmless, run of the mill substances later in life.

In this chapter, we will explore some of the more common autoimmune response diseases and their symptoms. For some readers, this may be the first time you have come across a dietary lifestyle book that is relevant and inclusive to your specific needs. For others, whose interests are rooted in the pursuit of overall health and wellness through an anti-inflammatory, autoimmune based diet, you are encouraged to read on. There may be one or two symptoms you have experienced in the past, that even on a subconscious level has prompted you into considering the Autoimmune Diet Protocol.

Autoimmune Hepatitis

When liver cells succumb to attack by white blood cells, they inflame and damage the liver, leading to one of the two forms of Autoimmune Hepatitis.

Type 1 Autoimmune Hepatitis is more widely seen in the medical community. Capable of affecting anyone at any age, it is seen mostly in female patients at approximately age forty-five.

Type 2 Autoimmune Hepatitis. Less common than Type 1, it is seen mostly in girls who are between the ages of two and fourteen.

With both types, symptoms present over several weeks, possibly months. The individual may also attend their general practitioner, citing feelings of being generally unwell, without any awareness of what might be the real cause.

Diagnosing and Treatment of Autoimmune Hepatitis.

Often, when the patient is receiving tests for reasons

other than presenting symptoms of hepatitis, the disease is diagnosed. Symptoms can go from minor to severe, including fatigue, joint, pain muscle pain, and a general feeling of being unwell. Loss of menstruation may also present. Persistent untreated inflammation causes liver damage,
including scarring of the liver, known as cirrhosis.

Provided the treatment is begun early; the outlook for this disease is favorable. With a treatment regimen followed by the patient, there is an excellent chance that the disease can be managed and brought under control.

Receiving treatment at the earliest possible stage will help regulate flare-ups, minimizing the likelihood of worsening the condition. Therapy over the long- haul can stifle further opportunity for the disease to develop. Over time, the damage to the liver may even be reversed. Aside from prescribed drugs, and other pharmaceutical measures, a diet specifically targeted at reducing inflammation may help with long term treatment plans.

Multiple Sclerosis (MS)

MS occurs when the central nervous system is attacked by the immune response system, compromising neurological responses, in other words, the ability for the spinal cord to transport messages from the brain to the rest of the body. The medical profession finds MS an astounding disease because of the severity and variety of ways it affects people.

People with MS commonly experience an unpredictable fluctuation of relapses and remissions. Attacks may come on suddenly, lasting for durations over several weeks. However, over time, each deterioration may intensify with less predictability and worsening of symptoms.

MS is in itself not fatal, but some people, because of the compromised immune system, are more susceptible to contracting other illnesses. Severe cases may sometimes result in vision loss and even paralysis.

Multiple Sclerosis is a chronic Autoimmune Disease that affects more than 2 million worldwide. Three times as many women as men suffer from the disease. The onset of the illness typically develops between the ages of twenty and forty.

Causes and Symptoms of Multiple Sclerosis

Genetics may play a role. If one parent has Multiple Sclerosis, there is a two to five percent risk the children will get the disease. Scientists believe that MS victims are born with a susceptibility to react to specific unknown environmental triggers adversely.

There has been a noticeable pattern of increased cases of MS sufferers in countries further from the equator. In places such as Northern Europe, scientists accept that exposure to lower levels of sunlight may play a role. Epidemiologists are therefore considering a possible correlation between Vitamin D, or lack of it, and the proper functioning of the immune system.

Viruses are known to cause inflammation. Researchers are also looking into the possibility that an infection may trigger the onset of MS in patients. Both the measles virus and human herpes virus-6 is under scrutiny.

Chronic fatigue is one of the most debilitating symptoms of this disease. MS-related fatigue occurs daily, worsens as the day goes on, and is more severe than normal fatigue. It may be the most conspicuous symptom in a person who otherwise has minimal signs.

Lack of coordination of muscle movement (ataxia), balance and functioning of the arms and legs are affected. Chronic back and muscle pain can result from simply walking. Sudden involuntary movements in all parts of the body is also a common sign.

Cognitive dysfunction is also prevalent among long term sufferers of MS. Notably, around half of the people with this disease demonstrate a decreased ability to concentrate, process information, and remember simple things.

Major depression is another condition of the disease. The stress of MS is known to alter moods to include increased irritability, unpredictable mood swings, and sometimes bouts of uncontrollable crying and laughing.

Altered sensory sensations to the skin like numbness, pins, and needles, tingling and tightness, and sharp stabbing pain are also present in some cases of MS. Eyes are sometimes affected by the disease. When the optic nerve has become inflamed, there is a potential for blurred vision, double vision, and uncontrolled eye movement. Continence problems, involving bladder incontinence, diarrhea, and constipation, are a difficult issue associated with this condition.

The importance of vitamin D, as noted earlier, may play an essential role in helping our immune systems function and support already compromised immune disease issues over the long term.

Celiac Disease

Celiac disease happens when wheat, oats, and other proteins such as grains cause the immune system to become inflamed. This protein is known as gluten. In some people, the consumption of gluten makes the immune system believe it is under attack and responds by producing inflammation, aggravating the inside of the small intestine.

The intense reaction to protein within the body results in damage to the interior of the bowel. When this area becomes inflamed, it is not possible for nutrients from food to become absorbed by the small intestine due to a flattening of projections along with the interior of the bowel.

Symptoms of Celiac Disease

Subsequent damage to the intestines can cause diarrhea, loss of energy and tiredness, loss of weight, feelings of sickness, and abdominal bloating.

Many people living with Celiac Disease are not even aware they have this issue! In fact, less than twenty-five percent are correctly diagnosed, leading to long term suffering and low nutrient absorption issues. However, long term damage to the intestines may take several years to present before the appropriate diagnosis is finally made clear to the patient.

Unfortunately, while not in itself, life-threatening, without the appropriate treatment, over time, any damage to the intestine may result in a worsening of symptoms due to increased inflammation. Many of those dealing with Celiac Disease may have other conditions that are presenting outside of the digestive tract.

Other problems such as anemia, loss of bone density, itching, and even damage to dental enamel have been known to present as symptoms worsen.

Complication Relating to Celiac Disease

Eventually, damage and the result of long-term inflamed tissue means the body is not able to provide sufficient absorption of the critical nutrients needed to maintain a healthy body. In extreme cases, this may result in malnutrition.

A body incapable of absorbing enough bone-building calcium and vitamin D may result in a weakening of bone connective tissue. In adults, this may present as osteoporosis, while in children, a softening of the bones in children, also known as rickets, may present. In young women of child-bearing age, calcium and vitamin D deficiencies have the potential to result in fertility complications and even miscarriage.
Celiac Disease can make life a misery, producing abdominal pain and diarrhea even after eating dairy products. Even a small amount of dairy provides a similar response to traditional lactose intolerance symptoms due to long term damage in the small intestine.

Given a chance to heal, significant damage to the small bowel may reverse, allowing for the consumption of dairy foods once again. However, for some, this may not be the case. For those people, they may remain lactose intolerant for an indefinite period.

A diet free of gluten is recommended for this Autoimmune Disease, to prevent further flare-ups and damage. Nowadays, gluten-free products are easily found in your average supermarket, making it possible to maintain a gluten-free dietary lifestyle.

Inflammatory Bowel Disease (IBD)

This disease is a generalized term for conditions presenting as an intense inflammation of the gastrointestinal area of the body. When the immune system functions correctly, it attacks organisms such as bacteria or viruses to protect the body. IBD is the result of a defective immune system, responding to environmental triggers that cause inflammation and damage to the intestines.

Inflammatory bowel disease is not a progressive condition and does not necessarily get worse over time. The severity of symptoms varies from time to time and person to person. Flare-ups of symptoms often seesaw from mild to severe and back to mild again, while others may experience quite long periods of remission. Sometimes months or even years elapse between flare-ups.

IBD interferes with the body's normal functions. When the disease is treated, controlling inflammation, most people can enjoy a relatively normal life. If left untreated, it can be debilitating and sometimes lead to severe complications.

The treatment goal for Inflammatory Bowel Disease is to control inflammation, relieve symptoms, and correct nutritional deficiencies.

Risk Factors of Inflammatory Bowel Disease

Inflammatory Bowel Disease may be diagnosed at any age; however, most people who develop inflammatory bowel disease do so before the age of thirty, although some do not contract the disease until they are fifty or sixty. Studies have shown that the risk of developing the condition is higher for people who have a close relative, such as a parent, sibling, or child with IBD.NSAID's may aggravate IBD, producing flare-ups, so it is best to avoid them when following an Autoimmune Diet Protocol.

Ulcerated Colitis and Crohn's Disease

Probably the most widely known of the inflammatory bowel diseases are Ulcerative Colitis and Crohn's Disease. In Ulcerative Colitis, the top layers within the intestinal lining become inflamed. With Crohn's Disease, however, the inflammation positions itself broadly throughout the entire wall of the intestine. For both diseases, however, the treatment is very similar.

Symptoms and Complications Common to Both

Symptoms common to both Crohn's disease and Ulcerated Colitis are primarily associated with low energy levels, a decrease in appetite, pain, and cramping of the abdominal region, blood in the stool, and even slow growth in children.

During periods of flare-ups for both diseases, there is an increased risk of developing inflammation of the eyes and skin lesions and other disorders, including arthritis, and an increase in the risk of blood clots. Side effects of some medications prescribed for inflammatory bowel disease may pose a small risk of developing high blood pressure and osteoporosis.

Rheumatoid Arthritis

Arthritic diseases commonly identified to most of us as pain and heat in the joints is caused by inflammation in the areas of wrists, ankles, knees, shoulders, and the other regions of frequent *wear and tear* use. People with this progressive disease go through times of higher activity or flare-ups, followed by times of stability or remission when the inflammation and pain either decrease in the severity or completely disappear.

Although this disease can strike at any age, the onset is most common between the ages of twenty-five and fifty-five.

Symptoms, Complications, and Management of

Rheumatoid Arthritis

The most common symptom of rheumatoid arthritis is tender, swollen joints; it is usual for both sides of the body to be affected by the disease. This painful joint disease typically starts in the joints surrounding the fingers, toes, and feet. As the disease progresses, the pain and swelling often spread to the ankles, wrists, hips, shoulders, knees, and so on.

When the lining of the membranes become damaged, the inflammation thickens the synovial membrane. Eventually, the cartilage and bone within the joint are destroyed.
Sometimes when the tendons and ligaments stretch and weaken, the joint gradually loses its shape and alignment.

Sleeping difficulties, because of pain, increase the persistent fatigue, which is a common condition of this disease. Medication for rheumatoid arthritis and the disease itself can further impair the immune system, leading to an increased risk of infection.

There is an increased risk of experiencing Sjogren's Syndrome, this disease, results in a reduction of moisture in the eyes and mouth. There is also a higher risk of inflamed and scarring of the lung tissue, which can lead to progressive shortening of the breath.

If rheumatoid arthritis has affected the wrists, it can lead to carpal tunnel syndrome. This syndrome causes inflammation and compression of the nerves serving the large motor skills associated with the hand and fingers. In more advanced and untreated cases, the arteries of the heart become hardened, leading to blockage, and ultimately inflaming the protective sac enclosing the heart.

Aside from exercise and rest, a diet rich in dark red vegetables and fruits such as black cherries and pomegranates may help. Scientists are learning that the compounds found in these fruits and vegetables may reduce inflammation and, over time, produce noticeable results.

Causes of Rheumatoid Arthritis

Genes do not cause rheumatoid arthritis. However, scientists believe that some people are more susceptible than others to environmental factors. Infection, viruses, and bacteria it is thought could be some of the factors that can trigger the onset.

It is thought that smoking increases the risk for people who, due to genetic factors, have are more likely to develop the disease than others without any predisposing genetic factors.

Systemic Lupus Erythematosus

Lupus, a difficult to diagnose Autoimmune Disease, lacks a single diagnostic test.
Signs and symptoms that closely mimic other medical conditions complicate the issue. Many tests may be needed to help rule any similar conditions that have similar symptoms.

What Is the Cause of Lupus?

Our immune system identifies and attacks foreign bodies, such as bacteria and viruses, to keep us healthy. For reasons not fully understood, our immune cells can reprogram and attack our cells and tissues, causing autoimmune diseases.

What triggers the autoimmune system to cause lupus is not known. Scientists believe that either environmental factors or genetics, or more likely a combination of both, are generally responsible. This combination of genetic predisposition and an external triggering event seems familiar to all expressions of autoimmune disease.

Potential triggers include sunlight, infection, and medication. Some blood pressure and anti-seizure medications, as well as antibiotics, have also been triggers, adding further complications to those dealing with the disease.

No two cases are exactly alike. The symptoms may appear suddenly, or in some cases, develop slowly. Symptoms can be mild or severe, temporary, or permanent. The disease is characterized by periods where the symptoms are highly active or *flare-ups*, and times of minimal or no symptoms, also known as *remission*.

Signs and Symptoms of Lupus

There are many symptoms of lupus. They vary significantly from person to person. It is, however, improbable that one person will experience all the possible symptoms.

The development of an unexplained low-grade fever is a sign of inflammation in the body. This fever is a classic symptom of lupus. Lupus is a disease that causes tissues in the body to become chronically inflamed. Joint and muscle pain is common for many people living with lupus. Itching, nausea, and swelling of the legs may indicate associated kidney damage.

Generally speaking, most individuals managing their lupus symptoms are likely to engage in what most people would recognize as a *healthy* life. However, there are variables and may ultimately rest on the severity of the disease and how committed the individual is to an overall healthy lifestyle, to include dietary modifications as recommended by their health care professional.

In conjunction with a medical professional, the Autoimmune Diet Protocol may help the conditions looked at in this chapter. It is never a bad idea to eat healthfully; however, when it comes to eating for specific immunity issues, even the humble tomato can raise an inflammatory response. Beans and nuts are full of healthy fats, can also create flare-ups for those managing autoimmune issues. In other words, it is not enough to follow a Mediterranean Diet, or even the much-lauded Paleo Diet, despite its close similarities to the Autoimmune Diet Protocol.

Healthy living and a healthy lifestyle have been demonstrated time and again to offer positive relief and benefits to most people suffering from illness and disease regardless of the projected outcome or the condition itself.

Closing this chapter out is a list of activities, a *to-do* list of sorts, designed to make you aware of some of the changes you might consider making both in your lifestyle and your diet.

Later, we will look at the benefits of supplements, exercise, and meditation, but for now, read on below and consider it a primer of sorts.

Next, we are going to look at the kinds of food we are allowed to eat, in addition to the food we are not allowed to eat, to include the order by which we reintroduce these foods into our diet. As always, we will need to remain mindful of any irritation or flare-ups once these foods are reintroduced. In the meantime, look at the list below and choose one or two things you can do right now today.

- Get enough sleep: Aim for between eight and ten hours per night, seven hours if you are an older adult since older adults often need less sleep.

- Manage stress: As we have seen, reducing our response to stress is so important when it comes to reducing flare-ups. Consider what stress-inducing events can you slide out of your life for good? What daily activities can you incorporate into your life to help manage any stress levels you are experiencing right now?

- Exercise: Even going for a walk has excellent health benefits. If you can exercise at a higher intensity, go for it! If not, that is okay too. Often, being outside in nature is a great stress reliever, with the bonus of taking care of our bodies also, through a walking activity.

- If you can walk or head to the gym with a friend, that can help you stay on target, with the added benefit of maintaining positive social interactions. Find out what works best for you and what you enjoy best. When you engage in activities you enjoy, studies show you are more likely to stick at it!

- Keep up those social connections! Even though there may be days when you just do not feel like it, even a ten-minute chat on the phone to a friend can offer great pick-me-up benefits. Just make sure you call or have coffee with an upbeat friend!

- No negative Nellie's! Negative people steal our energy, leaving even the most optimistic and healthiest among us, tired and drained. Take time to cultivate good quality friendships and relationships that make you laugh through the tough times; it will be worth the effort.

Chapter 3: Food Choices and Food Reintroduction

As with any diet, half the battle is knowing *what to eat* versus *what not* to eat. As we have already learned, following the Autoimmune Diet Protocol means following a strict, restrictive diet. For the full benefit to be realized, the protocol must be followed as closely as practicably possible for it to work.

In this chapter, we will look at the foods we can eat, the foods we are not allowed to eat, and the order with which to return some of those foods into our dietary lifestyle.

Some of us, on completion of the diet, may find we no longer want to include certain foods back into our meal plans. We may find that adding bread, for example, results in an inflammatory response, to the extent where it affects our moods. The gut and brain connections are not always considered when we reach for the typical diet and weight loss solution.

Most diets focus on losing weight through restricted calories, with varying degrees of success, depending on the food and the ability to stick with it. It will be helpful to remember that on this diet, the goal is to reduce inflammation in the body for overall health benefits, not weight loss per se. Of course, with any calorie restriction, weight loss usually follows.

It may be helpful also to consider that remaining on a restrictive calorie diet may not be the best solution in the long term. For some, depending on the autoimmune disease, a restrictive calorie diet may be harmful in the long run. The goal instead is to discover what foods you can eat going forward beyond the diet and which ones are best left out of your diet entirely. This may be different for many people. Autoimmune disorders, as we have seen, come in many shapes and sizes, with various treatments depending on the disease being managed.

Tackling the Autoimmune Diet Protocol- General Guidelines

• Aim to consume a minimum of six servings of vegetables each day. Ideally, if you can, try for nine servings. A full spectrum of vegetable colors is great to aim for, if possible.

• Eat many essential fatty acids. Consume healthy amounts of Omega 3's.

• Eat lots of food that supports healthy flora in the gut. Kampuchea, a fermented drink, maybe a good choice also.

• Don't wait to get hungry before eating! You may become hypoglycemic. Eat enough fats and protein to sustain your energy needs.

• Low blood glucose can cause energy crashes. Make sure you eat frequently enough to prevent low blood glucose.

• Drink. Drink and drink some more! Remain hydrated throughout the day by drinking plenty of water. Add electrolyte powder to your water if you need to, especially if you are working out. Staying hydrated also helps your body register as *full*, making you less likely to reach for the junk food.

• Steer clear of foods on the *Foods to Avoid* list. If you are to remain healthy and prevent flare-ups on while on the diet protocol, it is essential to remember that even the smallest portion of these foods may make you feel ill or affect your mood swings to the negative.

> • *KEY TIP...Seek support from friends and family members. Let them know you are going on this diet in the hope of feeling better and leading a healthy lifestyle. A little understanding and support from those closest to us can go a long way toward our success.*

•Monitor your blood sugar symptoms. By maintaining your healthy blood sugar, you will be able to recognize which foods trigger symptoms. If you do not already have one, you might be able to purchase a blood sugar monitor from your local pharmacy for a reasonable cost for this diet.

• The eliminating and reintroducing phase is meant to support the reduction in inflammation at the elimination phase. Ask the healthcare professionals on your immune management team for advice on how best to approach the reintroduction of key ingredients into your system.

Foods you can Eat

Most organic vegetables are available for this diet. Try to incorporate the best variety as much as possible; this includes the color spectrum of vegetables:

- arugula
- asparagus
- beetroot
- dark green leafy vegetables rich in Vitamin A
- bok choy
- broccoli
- red cabbage
- zucchini
- squash
- rhubarb
- carrots, purple and traditional orange
- cauliflower, rich in Vitamin C
- celery
- chives
- cucumbers
- mustard greens
- olives

- onions
- garlic, a fabulous natural anti-inflammatory
- leeks
- lettuce
- kale, rich in Vitamin A
- water chestnuts
- parsley
- radish
- spinach
- sweet potatoes
- yams
- watercress
- shallots,
- broccoli and kale are not considered detrimental to thyroid function, ask a medical professional if you are unsure.

Good quality cuts of meat, to include:

- beef
- pork
- wild game if available.
- chicken
- lamb
- bison
- turkey

If at all possible, select hormone-free and antibiotic-organically raised meat.

Organ meats and offal are also a great choice as they provide essential nutrients, fats that are healthy, and high in key amino acids. These include:

* heart
* tongue
* liver
* bone broth. Rich in glycine.
* kidney

Fish and shellfish are other options. Providing, of course, that you are not allergic! Select cold-water fish that is ocean-caught such as:

* low mercury fish with high-fat content.
* Swordfish
* Be careful with tuna-fish as sadly; it has a very high mercury content.

Fats from both animal sand fish are hugely important. The good fats are high in anti-inflammatory support:

* pasture-raised red or white meat
* grass-fed livestock
* cold-water fish, high in healthy fat
* olive oil, avocado oil, and Omega 3 supplements make sure they are low in mercury.

Low sugar content fruits:

- berries
- cherries
- apples
- plums
- peaches
- apricots, rich in Vitamin A
- avocado, rich in Vitamin E, and other skin-loving nutrients.
- grapefruit
- pears
- lemons

Consumable mushrooms are packed with essential micronutrients and are great for most people. However, check with your doctor for your particular medical or immune requirement.

Look out for the following fermented foods. Many of these are now readily available either on-line or at your local supermarket.

- kimchi,
- kombucha
- pickled ginger
- fermented cucumbers
- sauerkraut
- coconut yogurt
- coconut milk kefir

- Kefir is a form of cultured milk and helps support healthy bacteria in the lining of the gut
- water kefir

Noodles:

- Shirataki yam noodles
- AVOID any noodle that contains soy.

Cook with herbs and spices for added salt-free flavor in your meals:

- basil
- turmeric
- mace
- lemongrass
- coriander
- cilantro
- parsley
- cinnamon
- clove
- garlic
- ginger
- oregano
- rosemary
- sage
- sea salt
- thyme
- mint

- saffron
- horseradish

Avoid black pepper as it is a reintroduction item. Stave off iodized salt unless you're dealing with an iodine mineral deficiency.

It is permitted to consume vinegar products while on the Autoimmune Diet Protocol, however, check with your doctor if you have a condition that precludes the following varieties of vinegar and alcohol:

- apple cider
- avoid grain-based vinegar, rice, and distilled white vinegar.
- champagne
- red wine
- sherry
- balsamic
- coconut

Consuming good quality tea is also beneficial. Black teas are high in flavonoids which are natural anti-inflammatory qualities:

- black tea
- green tea
- white tea
- yerba mate tea
- assorted caffeine-free herbal teas

If you have adrenal fatigue, then avoid caffeine products.

Other food items or ingredients you can consume in moderation are:

- fructose, present in fruit and very starchy vegetables
- pomegranate
- molasses
- syrup
- honey
- dates
- date sugar
- unrefined cane sugar.
- Be careful with sugars since each person has a unique tolerance level.

Green beans and snow peas are possible for some; however, this may depend on sensitivity. If you are not sure, then you may wish to leave this out. Coffee may contain gluten contaminants, so be careful there.

Reintroducing Foods

Based on the process of eradication and food reintroduction, the Autoimmune Protocol Diet eliminates and also reintroduces a variety of food that may cause inflammation. Once the elimination is complete, and noticeable changes have occurred, then it is possible to begin the reintroduction phase.

This phase, however, is very exact and requires time and patience, making it possible to rule out reactivity.

Timing on the reintroduction of food depends on the individual. Monitor the reintroduction of food items until you become aware of a significant improvement in your symptoms and feelings of wellbeing. This may be as few as thirty days; for others, it may take as long as a full year, depending on the severity of your autoimmune deficiency issues.

Unraveling the repeating cycle of inflammation cycles lurking beneath your symptoms means the reintroductions mustn't be rushed. If you start reintroductions while you are still presenting sensitivity or allergic symptoms, it will be impossible to really understand whether a particular type of food that has been reintroduced is causing a reaction. If this is the case, unfortunately, you will end up starting all over again.

Stress levels, quality of overall sleep, our overall activity levels, intake of nutrients, all affect our reactions to foods as do genetics, and other underlying health issues if there are any present. In other words, once you start reintroductions, you will have to monitor for reactions closely. Sometimes, at the point of the reintroduction of symptoms begin to return. If this happens to you, it will mean you have to refrain from eating that food item, possibly indefinitely.

Reintroduction rules summarized:

1. Choose food items you wish to put back into your system. Consume several times, no more than three, and carefully monitor.
2. For the first time, eat no more than a half teaspoon. Wait between ten to fifteen minutes for a reaction.
3. If any signs of an adverse reaction happen, it is best not to consume that food again.
4. If no symptoms eat a whole teaspoon of the food. Once again, wait between ten to fifteen minutes, monitoring for signs.
5. If you are still without symptoms, eat a larger piece.
6. Wait three hours for any further signs of a reaction.
7. If, once again, there are no symptoms, eat the appropriately sized portion that you would typically eat.
8. Wait before consuming this food for about one week. At this point, monitor for symptoms.
9. If there aren't any symptoms within several days, then the food may be safe for you to continue eating.
10. Consume some of the food each day for the following week. Food reactions usually arrive in two forms; a strong response to a reintroduced food will leave little doubt as to the cause. A slower reaction building over time, becoming clear later. If, after the week, you are not experiencing any reactions at all, then that food is most probably okay for you to consume in the

long term, and you can now reintroduce another food item on the list into your diet.

Symptoms can arrive in the following ways, some of which you may be familiar with already, in which case you will immediately become aware of the reaction:

- upset stomach
- changes in mood
- tiredness and low energy
- pain
- problems getting to or staying asleep
- foggy brain
- skin irritations or rashes.

Following this diet protocol can take an incredible amount of time and patience; however, it is worth the time it takes. Understanding your unique inflammatory response to the food you consume will help in your long-term wellness goal.

PLEASE NOTE: If you have a response to a food reintroduction, wait till those symptoms are gone before continuing to further reintroductions. On how best to handle reintroductions correctly? Consult with your family or specialist doctor.

Negative Responses to Dairy, Eggs and Other Suspects

Some types of food may generate a negative response than others. Ideally, begin with food lowest on the list, ending with the most popular products. The appropriate method of reintroduction is:

Egg yolks, the yolks are tolerated by most people. It is the egg whites that have the highest level of intolerance. Soy protein used in some poultry feeds may be transferred to eggs, resulting in an intolerance.

Introduce seeds and nuts just one item at a time. Make sure the seeds and nuts are not soaked in oils or roasted as this can make the natural oils in the seeds and the nuts turn rancid.

With dairy, begin with grass-fed ghee before moving on to butter, goat yogurt or kefir, milk, and then cheese, before finally moving on to cow's milk. It is essential to consume these food items in this order because the raw enzymes in dairy make it comparatively easy to digest. Butterfat being more tolerable than the casein and lactose found in the other items.

If you have an inflammatory response, nightshades come last of all in the reintroduction phase. Because these mostly top the list of popular food intolerances for anyone dealing with immunity diseases, it takes more time to continue with these reintroductions and even longer for your immune response system to calm down. Settle down. Reintroduce no more than one vegetable at a time. Be prepared for one or more reactions.

Tomatoes, peppers, eggplant, and even potatoes form part of the nightshade family. For many with gut irritation and sensitivity, the lectins, saponins, and capsaicin found in these food items may worsen the condition.

It is best not to consume the following items:
- Tomatoes
- NSAIDs(these anti-inflammatory drugs have the opposite effect on the inflammatory system in some people)
- Gluten protein found in grains.

Your health history will determine on reintroducing other foods back into your diet. ***Legumes and grains*** contain high levels of protein. Lectins are known to degrade the barrier of the gut, adding to gut inflammation. Hauled off into the bloodstream, they stick to leptin and insulin receptors through the wall of the intestine. For some people, these receptors cause both insulin and leptin resistance due to long term desensitization.

Seeds and nuts are arguably highest among the allergens known to affect those with food sensitivities. A leaky gut stemming from the fiber in both nuts and seeds frequently occurs in those dealing with food sensitivities. Aside from some of the catastrophic allergic reactions to nut allergies, notably peanut, it may be best to avoid nuts altogether. An allergy to nuts is not uncommon in individuals, and it increases the chances of developing sensitivities and food allergies. One is ready to establish whether there exists a sensitivity by removing nuts and seeds during the removal stage.

Dealing with Subconscious Beliefs about Food

This diet is fraught with triggers for those fighting weight loss problems or enjoying the deliberate deprivation of food. In such cases, support may be needed for the relationship between the subconscious beliefs about your entire body, eating, and food. Lots of people are surprised to find that obsessions and cravings with food decrease or vanish as soon as they eliminate reactive foods and stabilize blood sugar.

Sugar and Scaling Back Inflammation

Inflammation affects millions of people around the world and is a precursor to many more serious diseases and health problems. One of the biggest culprits is sugar. Over the past fifty years, the food we eat has changed significantly, containing high levels of ingredients processed with salt and sugar.

As a result, obesity has reached epidemic proportions. Waistlines have increased and, losing weight can be very difficult. During the last twenty years, the rates of Type II Diabetes has increased. With predictable results, more people are now dealing with joint inflammation and an overall sense of aches and pains.

Substances such as high fructose corn syrup and other sugar substances not only spike blood sugar levels but also suppress our immune system. Once our immune system is down, as we have seen, the door to inflammation is opened.

Sugar is highly addictive, too, making giving it up or cutting it down even more difficult. Yet, if we are suffering from inflammation, cutting down our intake of sugar or eliminating it from our diet should be the first step we undertake. It is so effective that we will likely feel better within a few days to a week. For example, blood sugar levels spike when we consume a donut coated with powdered sugar. These spikes occurs when sugar hitting our bloodstream prompts a sudden release of insulin. Over time, if this continues to happen, these sugar spikes cause the body to become insulin resistant. In extreme cases, diabetes will occur.

Excess insulin stores as fat, resulting in weight gain, and the beginning of insulin insensitive. When our blood sugar levels are high, our joints, lungs, skin, and other organs are adversely affected, leading to health issues and inflammation.

So, what about artificial sweeteners? Despite the marketing hype about these artificial sweeteners being beneficial, the truth of the matter is that artificial sweeteners are worse than sugar. They are far more toxic and prevent the brain from receiving signals when our stomach is full. Consequently, we end up eating more than necessary, gaining excess weight.

You may wish to look for natural sugar alternatives such as stevia, honey, or pure maple syrup. Even cold fruit can satisfy a sweet tooth. Note, however, that even with these natural sugars, the body can still experience a blood sugar spike. However, it will not be as detrimental as what you would get with refined sugars.

As part of your Autoimmune Diet Protocol, begin a food journal and write down what you eat daily. Aim to make little and steady progress as you eliminate unnecessary foods from your diet.

Carbs and Inflammation.

When people think of foods that cause inflammation, they often think of sugar, sodas, artificial sweeteners, etc. Yet, nobody wonders about the white bread that comes with their hot dog. Or the white rice that accompanies their takeout.

These simple carbohydrates found in white bread, white rice, and white pasta are converted to a fast release compound known as glucose, also known as sugar, which, as we have seen, contributes to inflammation in the body to include the joints.

Eliminating carbohydrates from your diet, however, is not recommended. The body needs carbs to function well, but it is the slow release complex carbohydrates that your body needs for energy that should be the focus of your carbohydrate consumption.

These complex carbohydrates include vegetables, fruits, and grains. These are rich in fiber and are not high on the glycemic index. Green leafy vegetables, lentils, beans, peas, sweet potatoes, carrots, bananas, rice bran, cauliflower, barley, broccoli, bran, and whole-wheat bread are excellent sources of carbohydrates.

It is important to remember, however, that while on the Autoimmune Diet Protocol, some of these complex carbohydrates may be off theo list of foods you can consume. In some cases, depending on your particular Autoimmune Disease treatment protocol, you may not be able to eat some of these foods at all. It is essential, therefore, to refer to your treatment and dietary plan that you have with your medical practitioner.

That said, having as broad a mix of them as possible in your diet will mean you get sufficient soluble and insoluble fiber in your diet. When you are on an anti-inflammatory diet, ideally, about forty percent of your intake should be made up of complex carbs'. The remainder will be proteins and fats.

By consuming grains and vegetables, you will feel full much faster; beyond that, these are slow-digesting carbs meaning you will not feel hungry for quite a while. Your blood sugar levels will stabilize, and you will also be less likely to gain weight. Your body will shed the excess pounds and start feeling healthier. Losing weight is one of the best ways to reduce inflammation. The pressure on your joints will ease up, and you will be able to move more quickly.

Besides reducing your intake of refined sugar, cutting down your consumption of processed and simple carbs will be the next best thing that you can do to arrest your inflammation and slowly eliminate it.

Chapter 4: Supplements for Immunity

Our bodies are constantly at work coping with the damage of environmental toxins, intolerances to food, and diets high in inflammatory foods. It is essential, therefore, to support levels of immune-boosting nutrients in the body to minimize the damage taking place within our body.

In this chapter, we will look at several vital supplements that can help maintain a healthy immune system and may be useful to consider while engaging in the food restrictive Autoimmune Diet Protocol.

Do Supplements Work?

Supplements can have a beneficial effect on the body, especially when the body is going through a stressful time, or you are not able to obtain enough of the viral nutrients from fresh, high-quality food. Supplements are a personal choice and are not mandatory; however medical professionals are beginning to accept that supplements, as part of a healthy diet, maybe worth pursuing, at least in the short term, to monitor health benefits or positive changes.

Glutathione

Glutathione is a powerful antioxidant whose role is to support glutathione produced and recycled by the body. For those dealing with autoimmunity issues, including leaky gut, the role and support of glutathione become important. Glutathione aids in the regeneration of the blood and brain barrier, in addition to the gut lining. This support aids in the prevention of inflammation in the cells.

Glutathione's additional benefit is its role in the eradication of heavy metals and pollutants within the system. In this way, it makes a great anti-aging supplement!

Our diets are the primary source through which we maintain healthy glutathione sources. However, our poor diets, hectic lifestyles in addition to stressful circumstances, our body becomes deficient. The depletion of this antioxidant may result in disorders of the immune system, autoimmune flare-ups, and a permeable intestine, also known as Leaky Gut. Our chronically stressed lifestyle produces toxins within the body, making it a challenge to maintain glutathione. However, the supplement, S-acetyl glutathione, which more recently has become more affordable and readily available, may help manage Immune Disorders, through encouraging antioxidant support.

Dosage can start at around 1000mg a day generally. Higher doses may be required in neurodegenerative cases or advanced immune issues. Speak to your health care professionals if you think this supplement may work for your health situation.

Why is Glutathione Recycling Important?

Glutathione is a naturally occurring substance that serves as the body's antioxidant. With an antioxidant, the body can fight off free radicals that are formed by pollutants in the body as well as environmental exposure.

It is impossible to create glutathione for our bodies. We must get it from the food we eat, which helps our bodies produce the substance naturally. The extra glutathione we obtain from food is generally used in the body or used to supplement our bodies when we have depleted our glutathione stores.

When we consume too much of foods that are rich in calories, the body has to expend the stored energy in its waste products to maintain our body weight. By engaging in glutathione re-mineralization, the body can utilize the free glutathione we have to sustain the necessary energy. Excess energy is then used for maintenance.

With these excess wastes accumulating in the cells, damage to the cells and membrane that keeps them together occurs. Without their protective covering, the cells become susceptible to various diseases. Thus, any free glutathione we obtain from food is utilized for its benefit in maintaining the cell membranes, vital for your body's system operation.

Oxidative stress caused by free radicals can also damage cells. This is especially true for the cells in the mitochondria, which serve as the units that perform the necessary energy of our body; they are crucial for making our cells function as they do.

If the cells become damaged by oxidative stress, they cannot perform their functions properly. This could mean death for the cells, thus, requiring more energy from the body to keep the cells alive. Dead cells, also hang about after they have expired, thus slowing down the active, healthy cells.

Antioxidants do not work on their own; they are required for the proper functioning of the mitochondria as well as other cells. And importantly, are necessary for the ability of the body to repair itself after damage.

Increased levels of antioxidants result in increased amounts of glutathione that your body has available for use. Using up the free glutathione produced by the body also results in it becoming depleted of its antioxidants.

The Food you Eat Could be a Major Player in Boosting Glutathione Levels

Foods that support glutathione levels can help prevent oxidative stress. Oxidative stress is a natural process that occurs in our bodies when exposed to the oxygen molecules in our environment. The free radicals produced by this process then react with the proteins and other cellular parts of the body, damaging them to get rid of the debris.

Too much exposure to oxygen causes the body to create more free radicals than is necessary. This can be attributed to several factors, including a hectic lifestyle, lack of exercise, lack of sleep, unhealthy diet, and stress. All of these things combined can cause this reaction, which in turn depletes the body of its levels of glutathione. So, taking some sort of antioxidant supplements to help counteract this destructive reaction may play a vital role in supporting long term health goals. Of course, there are several different types of supplements on the market, but the best ones are going to be the nutrients we receive from our food.
In addition to over the counter antioxidant support, food plays a vital role in maintaining levels. This natural approach is always the preferred; however, for people managing autoimmune-related issues, this may be difficult, as some foods may be off-limits, either short or long term. Again, this may be something you wish to discuss with your health care provider.

In any case, banana shave a very high concentration of the essential vitamin A, also known as retinol, a potent antioxidant. Bananas also contain the antioxidant, vitamin C. Required for many functions; Vitamin C plays an essential role within the body. Additionally, it reduces the number of free radicals created by oxidative stress.

Antioxidants are not only good for the skin and the rest of the body, but they are also used for several diseases, including cancer, heart disease, and Alzheimer's disease. Additionally, the foods that support glutathione levels are believed to help relieve the symptoms of certain cancers.

Some of the most popular foods that support glutathione levels include fish, liver, strawberries, broccoli, black cherry, and nectarines. Red meat, eggs, and mushrooms are also considered to be high in this substance. On the other hand, it is recommended that people eat plenty of leafy green vegetables, which contain phytochemicals as well as other nutrients. The things that support glutathione levels can also help you feel healthier overall.

The benefits of the foods that support glutathione levels extend far beyond their role in increasing the levels of the hormone. These substances can also be useful in reducing free radicals produced by the body, thus increasing the ability of the immune system to fight off all types of illnesses.

Phytochemicals, found in foods such as broccoli, can provide a large amount of the glutathione that the body needs. Broccoli is also considered to be a great way to improve the health of the skin, which is one of the most common reasons that people use this herb to boost their immune systems. In addition, the phytochemicals in broccoli are said to help improve the skin's firmness and even the color!

L-glutamine and the Leaky Gut

L-Glutamine is a part of the body's immune system. It works to protect the brain and any other part of the body that it makes contact with a foreign molecules. Glutamine is an important part of many immune system functions that help to keep your immune system working well. When the immune system becomes depleted and cannot handle the strain, it is usually a precursor to inflammatory disorders such as Autism and Chronic Fatigue Syndrome and Leaky Gut. Those dealing with gut-related issues are often experiencing depleted levels of essential nutrients.

The cells need a source of energy. L-Glutamine helps the brain produce the essential enzyme ATP, the energy source for the brain cell functioning. When the cells are exposed to many environmental factors, they become much more susceptible to attacks from viruses, bacteria, fungi, and other toxins within the body. All of these toxins act to break down the walls that surround the cells, causing them to breakdown or leak, placing a strain on the functioning of this nutrient.

Probiotics

Probiotics play an essential role in our overall wellbeing. Stress and even poor hygiene practices can affect the good bacteria or probiotics in our gut lining. Antibiotics also have the potential to kill off this good bacterium, leaving us open to side effects such as Thrush.

Probiotics supplements, scientifically formulated to meet our nutritional are made from good bacteria or live organisms, making them suitable for digestion. Ideally, a good supplement will include Acidophilus, Lactobacillus, Bifid bacterium, and Bifid bacterium. These are the live organisms that help the human body digest food better. There are many forms of probiotics available, choosing one that contains all the probiotics should provide the overall support required.

Digestive Enzymes

Digestive enzymes are the building blocks of our bodies. As we live, the food we eat gets broken down in our mouth and goes through the system to be absorbed. The digestive enzymes are the link between the foods we eat and the raw materials which the body uses for its utilization.

The body has a great ability to break down the different substances it consumes. Digestive enzymes act as detectors. They immediately recognize certain things and convert them into the necessary nutrients the body needs. If the body does not have the required proteins, food will get broken down before it reaches the colon. When this happens, the body has not fully utilized the essential vitamins and minerals it needs, sending them to the various parts of the
body. Nutritional benefits are, therefore, limited. There are many types of over the counter digestive enzymes available, providing the same benefits as taking enzymes naturally through food. Digestive

supplements such as papaya, for example, do not have any adverse side effects and can be taken in supplement form with food or with pills, making this one of the easiest and acceptable supplements to take.

Vitamin D

The body produces Vitamin D in reaction to sunlight and is well known for its wide-ranging health benefits. Researchers also have discovered vital cells of the immune system are positively affected. These positive effects extend to Autoimmune Diseases such as Multiple Sclerosis.

Researchers have also discovered it affects critical cells within the immune system.
This key discovery may help us understand the way with which vitamin D regulates immune reactions implicated in autoimmune diseases such as Multiple Sclerosis.

Vitamin D, found in natural exposure to sunlight, has been found to reduce the impact of diseases as far-ranging as heart disease, arthritis, and even strokes. More recently, it has been noted in its effects on autoimmune diseases and the impact of viruses on the immune system.

Considering these studies, taking a vitamin D supplement might be worthwhile along with a nutrient-rich, anti-inflammatory diet.

Zinc

Insufficient zinc – a condition that affects as much as twenty-five percent of the world's population, has been found to alter the makeup of bacteria inside the intestine.

Studies have shown that physiological ailments and many diseases, including diabetes, depression, obesity, and cardiovascular diseases, have links to natural gut bacterial ailments.

Zinc, taken following professional guidelines, may be useful in playing a long-term role in maintaining both gut and mood health, especially in individuals dealing with Autoimmune Diseases.

Zinc and health are closely related. When there is an imbalance of the right kind of nutrients in the body, the body will respond with problems such as low energy, weak bones, depression, and other disorders. To get the proper amount of zinc, a person needs to eat a balanced diet that includes both animal and plant protein.

Zinc is also needed to improve the function of the brain and to help it produce a hormone called serotonin. Zinc makes serotonin and the other hormones in the brain more responsive to changes in the environment.

Zinc, too, is needed for maintaining a healthy immune system by helping the body's ability to produce substances that help it fight disease. While it can also help maintain body strength, it is most important to get enough if you want to keep your brain healthy.

Brain health has become one of the more prominent topics of discussion today. The brain is essential in performing all day-to-day tasks needed to maintain physical and mental health. It is the "working" part of the body, but it is the one part of the body that is most susceptible to age-related degeneration.

It is because of this that a healthy brain and gut are so crucial to overall health. By paying attention to keeping our mind healthy, we may find that the mind and bodywork together holistically and healthily.

Depression, we have seen throughout this book, may, in some people, be linked to the relationship between our gut and the chemical responses of our brain. This new, exciting revelation may mean it is possible to treat depression with more than medication. By understanding it as having a possible link to a weak immune response, and gut inflammation, new treatment options may become available.

An effective immune system is behind an efficient ability to heal from diseases, in addition to the ability to fend off disease, especially concerning cell regeneration. Cell regeneration has become an exciting field of study for brain health. It is among the areas of health research that is currently focusing on developing more effective treatments for brain and gut health. Researchers believe that improving the brain and immune system function will lead to better functioning of all other organs also.

Increased cell regeneration is critical to any success regarding boosting the immune system to help with healing. In particular, the brains of patients suffering from diseases like Alzheimer's or Parkinson's disease function worse than those who do not have those diseases. Researchers have discovered that the brain's immune system can actually become confused and inflexible after exposure to germs and toxins. This becomes yet another excellent reason why it is essential to look at the key nutrients we put into our diet for long term health and healthy longevity.

Zinc found in the building block of proteins has proven to be exceptionally important in maintaining brain health and in preventing the buildup of fats known to cause diseases such as heart disease and cancer. It is the easiest and one of the most affordable supplements to absorb, making it an excellent choice for anyone trying to combat the effects of a weak immune system.

Vitamin C

Vitamin C, also known as ascorbic acid, is a water-soluble antioxidant acting as a coenzyme in the production of vitamin E. Vitamin C also helps control the formation of free radicals. Free radicals are harmful molecules that are responsible for damaging tissues, DNA, and other cellular components. These harmful molecules attack cells, causing them to die off. One of the ways to reduce the effects of free radicals is by taking in Vitamin C supplements. Antioxidants protect the body from the harmful effects of free radicals. Because of this, it helps in lowering the risk of developing diseases such as cancer, heart disease, and even osteoporosis. Taking antioxidants has many benefits, and one of them is that they help in lowering the risk of cancer and improving the body fight against osteoporosis.

Vitamin C is found in fruits, vegetables, and many other food sources. Even if you don't eat a lot of fresh produce, you can still get enough Vitamin C through the consumption of cooked vegetables. Adding lemon to your greens and tomatoes to your fruit salads will help your body get more Vitamin C. Of course, you can also take Vitamin C supplements.

To understand the importance of Vitamin C, we need to understand the role of the immune system. It protects the body from bacteria, viruses, and other harmful substances. When the immune system gets weak, the body's defenses are vulnerable to attacks from these dangerous substances. Vitamin C, being an antioxidant, helps keep a healthy immune system.

Vitamin C also helps keep bones strong and healthy. The increased calcium levels due to Vitamin C in the body maintain strong and healthy bones. Eating plenty of fresh fruits and vegetables will ensure that you are getting enough vitamin C. Vitamin C is also found in protein, which is present in meat, fish, poultry, and eggs. If you can't consume Vitamin C in your diet, you can always take Vitamin C supplements. The main difference between Vitamin C supplements and Vitamin C that you eat is that the latter cannot be digested.

For this reason, you should know the difference between Vitamin C that you eat and Vitamin C that you take. This will help you determine which supplements are best for you. Many vitamin supplements nowadays contain the synthetic form of Vitamin C, such as Ascorbic Acid. Since the body can't digest it, Ascorbic Acid is a synthetic version of Vitamin C.

The Health Benefits of Vitamin C

Incorporating a daily dose of Vitamin C into your diet may have a wide range of benefits on the immune system. As shown below, its benefits may extend way beyond the common cold.

For those dealing with immune disorders, Vitamin C might be a worthwhile supplement to add, especially if your diet restricts certain foods or substances found in food, due to irritation of the gut and so on.

Colds, unfortunately, as miserable as they make us feel, do not have a cure. Thankfully, however, Vitamin C is a small but essential part of your immune system in preventing nuisance illnesses such as these. Autoimmune Diseases such as Multiple Sclerosis leave our overworked immune systems vulnerable to attack; stress, of course, being another contributor to lowered immune systems. Vitamin C helps the body to produce and use antibodies that fight off pathogens.

The benefits of taking Vitamin C for stroke prevention are impressive. Numerous studies have shown that this vitamin has a positive effect on the prevention of stroke.

Vitamin C is essential for maintaining good circulation, proper functioning of the cardiovascular system, and healthy red blood cell formation. Also, Vitamin C increases energy and helps to restore the body's strength. Another benefit of taking Vitamin C for stroke prevention is its ability to prevent damage to brain cells that can lead to stroke. For example, Vitamin C stops nerve fibers from being damaged, which is a known risk factor for stroke. Taking Vitamin C can also help reduce the occurrence of amyloidosis, a condition that is linked to Alzheimer's disease. All of these benefits of taking Vitamin C for stroke prevention are well documented in scientific research.

It is widely accepted that stress has an adverse reaction on the immune system, which, long term, may lead to viruses and other immune disorders.

Vitamin C has been shown to benefit the immune system of anyone experiencing stress through life challenges, work, and even lifestyle habits such as consuming excess alcohol and smoking.

The vitamin produces mood-enhancing neurotransmitters, such as norepinephrine, making them critical to the brain's proper functioning and long-term health. Overall, Vitamin C stimulates the white blood cells necessary in the fight against infections and viruses.

Food Sources of Vitamin C

An accessible list of Vitamin C rich foods and recipes includes the following easy-to-get produce:
- citrus fruits
- grapefruit
- papaya
- oranges
- watermelon
- banana
- kiwi fruit
- mango
- pineapple
- broccoli

Many fruits and vegetables contain Vitamin C. Fresh fruit, juices, and juices from cooked fruits are more easily digested than processed foods. It also takes longer for the fruits to digest, so they will be more nutritious. If you buy a cup of commercially prepared juices, make sure the label has the recommended daily dose of Vitamins C, and A. Watermelon, orange, kiwi, and mango are great sources of this C vitamin, so take the time to look at the ingredients.

Watermelon is an excellent source of Vitamin C; if it is freeze-dried and then made into cold press juice extractions, this type of melon is very nutritious. Bananas are also one of the best sources of Vitamin C. Its purple-tinged skin helps to inhibit the growth of bacteria that cause scurvy, an ailment that can cause weakness, cramps, confusion, and other severe symptoms.

The best way to get your daily dose of vitamin C is through your diet, as opposed to turning only to supplements. You should aim to eat at least nine servings of fruits and vegetables per day. This will give you the bounty of phytochemicals, vitamins, and minerals necessary in addition to a healthy dose of this Sunshine Vitamin.

Half a cup of fresh orange juice will help you reach your recommended daily allowance; however, adding the following food items may help keep things interesting. As always, though, make sure your unique sensitivity issues are taken into consideration first:

- One cup cantaloupe
- A single cup of tomato juice

- 1 medium-sized kiwi

- 1 cup cooked broccoli

- Half a cup of green pepper -Make sure this is cooked. Uncooked green pepper has a toxic effect on the body.

- Half a cup of red cabbage

Studies have shown a large number of adults in the US fail to consume enough Vitamin C, even though this is a relatively natural and easy vitamin to obtain.

Lack of Vitamin C, as we have seen, can lead to more than the common cold should the immune system be placed under stress. Stress, of course, weakening the immune system, making it susceptible to viruses, both common, in addition to the more serious such as pneumonia and bronchitis.

How Do We Get More Vitamin C?

The following tips may help you work more Vitamin C rich fruit and vegetables into your diet. They are easy to implement, and many of the ingredients are readily available at regular supermarkets.

Pre-prepare fruit and vegetable produce by cutting them up in advance and placing them in a lunch box before work. This way, you will have them handy when needed.

Fruits and grated vegetables can be incorporated into family dishes such as:

- meatloaf
- soups
- muffins
- brownies
- biscuits, and more.

Slice fresh fruit and freeze it as an alternative to sugary popsicles or ice cream. Frozen grapes, red or white, make a great treat on a hot day.

Supplement Considerations

The most significant source of any vitamin consumption and benefit is through obtaining the nutrient naturally. However, if you are taking or plan to take the supplement, the brief guide below might be of some assistance. As always, consult a medical professional if there are any pre-existing conditions whereby a Vitamin C supplement may not be appropriate.

- Nicotine products like smoking, and painkillers such as aspirin, oral contraceptives, illegal drugs, can all reduce the amount of Vitamin C in the human system. If these products are being taken by you or you are a smoker, you might want to discuss increasing intake.

- Avoid this supplement if you are taking Warfarin or any related prescription medication; in this situation, you should attempt to obtain your daily dose through the right food choices.

- Vitamin C is considered safe when obtained from supplements or food sources. Although the side effects are uncommon, in some cases, however, too much Vitamin C may result in a stomach upset. Adults can consume about two-hundred-fifty milligrams of Vitamin C, any more than that is passed out via the bladder.

- At times of extreme stress, to include illness, our body requires more Vitamin C than average. During these times, your health care professional may advise you to consume more Vitamin C than typical. This may be especially true for someone managing an immune deficiency

Health Risks from Deficiency

Some of the signs of vitamin C deficiency include frequent headaches, muscle aches, weakness, excessive tiredness, and blurred vision. The symptoms can also be confused with severe health conditions like heart disease or kidney disease. When you are diagnosed with either of these conditions, you will most likely be prescribed medication that will help alleviate your symptoms. If you are dealing with issues such as Leaky Gut, this inability to absorb Vitamin C nutrients will contribute to a deficiency of this vitamin.

One of the more common effects of Vitamin C deficiency is depression. According to many studies, failure to absorb the optimum amount of nutrients from their diet are more likely to develop depression. Aside from the fact that this nutrient is essential for healthy skin, hair, and nails, it can also help promote emotional stability. A lack of Vitamin C can lead to feelings of sadness, anger, anxiety, and even irritability.

The deficiency between Vitamin C and Arthritis are closely related. Both these disorders have one thing in common - joint pain. Therefore, it is a good idea to know the causes of vitamin C and arthritis.

Vitamin C is an antioxidant, which is essential for cell metabolism. When Vitamin C metabolizes cells, it can increase the energy production of the cells, which makes it is vital in preventing cellular damage. For this reason, Vitamin C is beneficial in Rheumatoid Arthritis. It helps in producing collagen, a substance that supplies bone structure. Collagen is essential for the normal functioning of joints. Vitamin C also helps in the formation of cartilage, cartilage helping to provide elasticity to

the joints, in addition to comfort via the collagen maintained via Vitamin C.
A deficiency of Vitamin C and Arthritis may be a sign of Rheumatoid Arthritis, a condition that can be acquired from several other diseases, including Autoimmune Diseases.

A deficiency of Vitamin C and Arthritis can be prevented by eating lots of fresh fruits and vegetables, such as the ones suggested earlier. Eat several servings of these fruits and vegetables every day. Avoid using supplements, unless specifically recommended by your doctor.

Poor Immune Function

Vitamin C and low immunity are two different things. Vitamin C is often confused with the immune system boosting substances like immune blockers, or probiotics. These substances help improve the immune system by making it stronger and more resilient. Vitamin C actually helps prevent the body from losing immune system strength and effectiveness.

Vitamin C and low immunity are probably best treated as different diseases, rather than as symptoms of the same condition. Many different things can cause immune system problems. A poor diet, fatigue, and stress are all known causes of weakened immune systems. If you are experiencing symptoms of a Vitamin C deficiency, or if you have an autoimmune problem, your immune system might be doing some of the jobs that the body's cells and tissues are not doing.

Foods that are high in raw, leafy vegetables are good sources of vitamin C. Fruits and vegetables are excellent sources of a wide variety of vitamins and minerals, including calcium, iodine, potassium, and iron.

Foods high in vitamin C are the best way to get your body the most out of what it needs to keep your immune system healthy. You should take the amount of Vitamin C that is recommended for you according to your recommended daily allowance. If you don't consume enough vitamin C, your body could develop an improper immune system and deficiency of vitamin C in your diet.

You should also stay away from foods that are high in sugar. Sugar triggers your body to make insulin, which then gives sugar to your cells. This sugar then leads to chronic inflammation and is also a contributing factor to low immunity. Get rid of the food sources of sugar substitutes, and you should improve your vitamin C levels and low resistance to viruses.

As we have seen throughout this book, we rely on our immune system to protect our bodies from disease. This may be influenced by our intake of minerals and vitamins, particularly vitamin C. There are many cells within our systems that need vitamin C to do tasks that are basic, so a deficiency reduces resistance against pathogens. Vitamin C lessens the severity and duration, in addition to the risk of disease of the disease, and keeps our body in prime condition.

Antibiotics, Can They Destroy our Immune System?

There are literally billions of bacteria both within and outside the human body. Some of these bacteria cause diseases and are considered pathogenic or disease-causing. The others are understood to be beneficial to the human body, living symbiotically within us. When we are prescribed antibiotics for an illness, we eradicate the good bacteria along with the harmful bacteria. Unfortunately, this may cause more disease than we started with.

This mainstream practice in the overuse of antibiotics may be driving the dramatic rise in inflammatory conditions. These inflammatory conditions include Type 1 Diabetes, Obesity, Allergies, Inflammatory Bowel Disease, and Asthma. Startlingly, over the years, many of these diseases have doubled, according to medical experts and immunological researchers.

We, by design, are "meta organisms," this means we have a lot of microbial organisms living on the various aspects of our body and within the body, particularly in the gastrointestinal area. There is good evidence to suggest that these healthy microbes are there to assist us. They help us derive energy from complex carbohydrates we cannot break down, and help us gain access to highly beneficial nutrients, such as vitamin K known for its blood clotting abilities. These healthy organisms also help us fight off viral infections, and it is now believed that they protect us from Autoimmune Diseases, Multiple Sclerosis being one of them.

Antibiotics and their Consequences

Without question, antibiotics are exceptional medications. They are implicated in the reason why we have a longer life span—from age sixty-three in 1940 to seventy-eight in those living today in the United States.

However, a major problem with the overuse of antibiotics is that the scientists screen out and eliminate drug-resistant organisms. The second big problem is that antibiotics change the microbial contents of those living on our bodies, which can adversely affect the immune system. One of the side effects of these medicines is the presence of yeast infections.

One study showed how the gut bacteria were affected by two prescribed courses of the medication ciprofloxacin; an antibiotic used quite commonly. Using the antibiotic resulted in profound and important changes in the presence of microbes within the lining of the gut that never fully recovered from being in their original state.

Other studies have demonstrated that changes within the gut bacteria, including the presence of organisms resistant to antibiotics, may remain compromised for up to three years, more in some cases.

Studies have also shown that the bacterium in our guts, also known as Helicobacter pylori, is related to inflammation within the stomach, stomach ulcers, and stomach cancer. This bacteria has lived within our guts forever; however, it is quickly disappearing from the gut area. Presently, there are only six percent of children in Europe and in the US that still have the microbe in their system.

Immune Signaling Systems

While these beneficial bacteria help our health, scientists still have no idea how they affect metabolism and immunity within our biological systems. Antibiotics can cause the presence of the bacteria known as Clostridium Difficile, which can also be present in healthy people. This bacterium can cause severe infections that may result in the inflammation and infections of the colon when the other beneficial bacteria have been killed off.

In studies of healthy, germ-free mice, it was discovered they are prone to getting infections by food poisoning bacteria. These food poisoning bacteria may cause severe cases of Salmonella when compared to those with average amounts of bacteria in their gut walls.

Research has revealed the presence of microbes
within our body makes for a complicated system. It
is this system; however, that keeps us healthy.
Certain gut bacteria are known to stimulate T cells, a
type of white blood cell capable of reducing or
promoting inflammation as part of our beneficial
immune response. This gut flora, when healthy and
not compromised by antibiotics, maintains a healthy
balance between the pro-inflammatory T cells and
the anti-inflammatory T cells. An imbalance,
however, can cause susceptibility to immune
diseases such as diseases of the bowel and Multiple
Sclerosis.

Immunologists maintain we need to more
judiciously deploy the use of antibiotics and develop
drugs targeting only specific bacteria. This will leave
the healthy bacteria unharmed. A deeper
understanding of probiotics may assist the immune
system by building up healthy bacteria following on
from the use of antibiotics. It is hoped that
probiotics will one day be used in tandem with
antibiotic prescriptions in order to help maintain
healthy bodily flora.

Are you enjoying this book? If so, I'd be really happy
if you could leave a short review on Amazon, it
means
a lot to me! Thank you.

Chapter5: Inflammation and Good Fats Versus Bad Fats

Many scientists and researchers continue to explore the question of what are good fats? One of the leading experts in this area of study is Dr. Richard Feinman, Ph.D., professor, and expert on biochemistry and aging.

There has been a lot of controversy over what is good or bad for you and your health. Are the so-called "bad" things actually healthy, or is it more important to focus on the good things?
In many respects, carotenoids are considered "good" because they are thought to be antioxidants. Antioxidants neutralize free radicals that cause cellular damage.

Carotenoids are concentrated in plants, fruits, vegetables, and seeds, such as carrots, spinach, and apricots. Carrot juice, made from ground carrots, contains high levels of carotenoids.

It has been known for decades that antioxidants have a protective effect on our bodies and those of animals. It has also been found that antioxidants can lead to cancer prevention and possibly even prevent tumor growth.

The antioxidant nutrients in fruits and vegetables help in many ways. Vitamin C, as we have already seen, helps us ward off colds and disease. Antioxidants help block inflammation, which may be one of the reasons why inflammation plays such a role in aging and cancer. That is a good thing, but it is also a tricky proposition, because our body produces inflammation and, although we can fight it, it will inevitably return after a while.

Our bodies produce inflammatory compounds called cytokines, and the molecules that bind to them, called interleukins, can help inhibit and repair damaged cells, tissues, and organs. We know that these cytokines can lead to inflammation when they attach to some cells to signal that those cells are malfunctioning, which results in that signal being passed on to a malignant cell and the formation of a tumor.

Inflammation is most common in those older adults who are managing an Autoimmune Disorder, such as Arthritis, Lupus, Diabetes, Multiple Sclerosis, and systemic Lupus Erythematosus. Inflammation is also known to be a factor in the development of many Autoimmune Diseases, including Rheumatoid Arthritis, Alzheimer's Disease, and Chronic Fatigue Syndrome.

Some of the common immune-related diseases that have been associated with inflammation and a lack of antioxidants are Osteoarthritis, Peptic Ulcers, Irritable Bowel Syndrome, Psoriasis, and Lupus. Some of these problems are made worse by long-term inflammation, while others only get worse if it is not treated with the appropriate medical therapies and diets such as the Autoimmune Diet Protocol. It is not just inflammatory diseases that can lead to autoimmunity, but it is also a known fact that most of the diseases of aging have a genetic component. There is no cure for most of these conditions; neither are the causes of autoimmune disorders fully understood. Therefore, it may be a good idea to get some form of antioxidant and anti-inflammatory supplements. The ones outlined in this book may provide a good starting point in the fight to help control autoimmunity and age-related immune deficiencies.

Eating foods that are high in antioxidants, such as dark green, leafy vegetables, avocado, celery, and nuts and low-fat dairy products is one way to get some good fats. However, if you are attempting to manage your Autoimmune Disease or disorder, check with your health care professional to make sure that the foods you are taking are not restricted food items that would cause a flare-up.

In this diet, especially with respect to the reintroduction of particular foods following the diet protocol, there will be many differences between those who are able to eat certain food items and those who cannot. It will all depend on individual needs.

Additionally, if you are restricted from eating, tomatoes, for example, in the case of diverticulitis, ask your health care professional if you may be able to supplement with lycopene, the antioxidant found in tomatoes.

The Difference between Good and Bad Fats

Many people wonder what the difference between good fats and bad fats is. It has been somewhat controversial at times as people argued against the possibility that good fats existed. However, as the body of research continues to grow, many people are now becoming increasingly educated on the subject of dietary fats. So, if you are wondering what the difference between good fats and bad fats is, here are a few things you should know.

When we eat foods that contain fat, the body converts these fatty acids into fuel to run our body. The energy is then stored as glycogen within our liver. If we eat a lot of high-quality food, the body has plenty of glycogen to store this energy for use later. This is one of the most important reasons for eating a diet rich in good fats.

The problem arises when you eat foods that contain very little fat yet are rich in carbohydrates. These foods are also referred to as "empty" calories. You can think of these as "good fats" that are digested and turned into energy, but because they contain many empty calories, the body is not able to use them to produce energy.

This is why so many people suffer from inflammation and other problems to include

arthritic joints. Many sufferers are eating a diet rich in "empty" calories and would benefit from a positive change to their diet.
Healthy fats contain mostly unsaturated fatty acids or the good fat that is digested by the body and converted into energy. When you are on a diet, you cannot eat the foods that contain those unsaturated fatty acids. Therefore, you might want to consider taking supplements containing healthy fats to include gamma linoleic acids such as borage oil and evening primrose oil. These fats are also capable of helping minimize the unhealthy inflammatory responses in the joints of arthritis suffers.

Excess insulin in the blood due to low nutrition, high sugar diet, as we have seen, causes several problems in the body. Therefore, most people who are diagnosed with diabetes are told to lose weight and are immediately placed on a restrictive calorie, but nutrient-rich diet.

In terms of nutrition, we need to start thinking about feeding the cells in our body, and not just feeding to fill our stomachs. This, while it may sound idealistic, is, in reality, what is necessary to take care of both the hunger and the nutritional intake needed. The challenge for many, however, is to find the right combination of healthy food capable of doing all the above. Additionally, we still need to satisfy our cravings as well.

It is also true that if you have a thyroid condition, you can be at increased risk for developing chronic arthritis. Many thyroid conditions are caused by too much of a hormone called cortisol; cortisol, as we will see a bit later, is produced by the adrenal glands when we feel under stress, or if we are anxious. This is a natural response, however, when cortisol levels are low, the immune system is weakened, and arthritis is an increased likelihood to develop.

As we begin to replace unhealthy foods with healthy foods, we may notice some definite differences in our symptoms. Some people report they have less pain in their joints after they have lost weight. Others claim this happens right away.

When it comes to the prevention of arthritis from occurring, the experts do not recommend supplements. Instead, they say that it is best to eat a healthy diet rich in fiber and other plant-based foods. Fiber is essential because it helps your body eliminate waste products and keep the colon clean.

However, in situations where a restrictive diet is necessary due to food sensitivities, it is worth asking your health care professional for a list of approved supplements. Having a sensitivity to certain food items does not mean that you do not need them. Antioxidants and the healthy fats found in a natural diet of real food have been proven to alleviate some negative immune responses. Attempting to help these nutrients find their way into your diet, therefore, may be beneficial both in the long and short term.

How do Good Fats Help with Autoimmune Diseases?

The relationship between good fats and leaky gut is only just being understood as they relate to autoimmune diseases. Oils, at least the healthy ones, are becoming more acceptable as a legitimate and healthy method of cooking the food we need to remain at optimum immune health. It is essential also to understand that, for the nutrients from the food we eat to be absorbed, we need a certain amount of healthy fat to assist in the absorption.

Leaky gut is caused by the hyperactivity of the immune system in the small intestine leaving small holes from which nutrients are then able to leak out, causing other abdominal issues. The upshot is your body's inability to digest the foods entering the body properly. This results in a buildup of harmful substances in the digestive tract. The symptoms of this condition include acne, fatigue, joint pain, depression, and other undesirable conditions. Researchers know that a diet rich in specific foods such as fruits, vegetables, whole grains, and nuts can go a long way in healing the Leaky Gut condition. However, other Autoimmune Disease that also results in a leaky gut means it can be challenging to pinpoint a one size fits all diet plan.

However, in general, terms, to create a diet that will treat leaky gut and associated ailments, researchers have turned to the use of supplements to add healthy fats and lauric acid to the diet. Olive oil and coconut oil being great sources of these fats. They not only supply essential vitamins and minerals but also provide the body with the right amount of lauric acid.

In addition, these oils, rich in beneficial Omega-3 Fatty Acids, which can assist the body tackle infections caused by viruses, bacteria, fungi, and parasites. Because these fatty acids work against the growth of these organisms, the body can kill off many of them.

Olive oil is also a known moisturizer used to treat dry skin, acne, and other similar conditions due to the presence of the anti-inflammatory presence of squalene. Squalene has recently gained attention not only as an anti-aging skincare ingredient but also in the treatment of cholesterol, and possibly even cancer, although there as yet there have not been any human trials. Either way, there is a growing appreciation for the anti-inflammatory properties of olive oil and its numerous health benefits.

 Also, it is a popular ingredient in gourmet foods because due to its comparatively pleasant taste compared to other oils.

With respect to coconut oil, although this particular oil is healthy for many people, it is still possible to develop problems when using it. For example, a reaction to peanuts and other nut products may result in an unpleasant response when using this particular oil. For those people, it might be best to avoid it altogether, opting for olive oil instead.

Allergies can be challenging to treat because they are not easily identifiable. This is one of the reasons why research continues to learn how to detect them and treat them. Of course, if you are allergic to peanuts, this means that you are unable to use this oil.
These oils can then be an excellent addition to your diet. Like anything else, though, if you want to experience all the benefits of these oils, you must make sure that you take in the right amounts of each one.

Five Disease Preventing Cooking Oils

We all love delicious food; this goes without saying. In fact, many of our favorite meals are prepared by frying with a small amount of oil. However, have you ever thought about the oil your food is prepared with? Just because the oil is vegetable-based, does not mean it is suitable for your overall health.

Luckily, there are some great cooking oils that not only help prevent health risks but support good health, especially heart health. These are edible oils that should be taken advantage of, as they can prevent disease and promote overall long-term health.

A word of caution, however, when cooking with oils. Not all oils are created equal. Check on the bottle to make sure the oil you are selecting can be used to the cooking temperature that you will need. Some oils, when heated, turn rancid, producing carcinogens, or free radicals, therefore, ruining any of the oil's health producing benefits. These carcinogens and free radicals can cause inflammation, with the potential to make a significant contribution to an inflamed gut!

Coconut Oil

What was traditionally considered "exotic," coconut oil is fast making its way back to being the premier choice for cooking. In recent years with a resurgence of interest, coconut oil has been heavily researched and found to be superior for daily use. Amongst its marked properties are:

- **Stability** - coconut oil is not liquid at room temperature, but rather a semi-solid. It can survive for months, even years when kept in an airtight container without going rancid and is therefore perfect for stored use.
- **Rich in Lauric Acid Lauric**, which has a marked effect on reducing cholesterol levels and is extremely favorable to overall heart health.
- **Rich in Medium Chain Triglycerides** - MCTs found in coconut oil can produce ketone bodies, compounds, which act as alternative energy sources to carbohydrates. This makes coconut oil especially helpful when trying to keep up energy levels on a low-carb diet. Increased energy levels can help improve weight loss.

Olive Oil

An exceedingly popular oil, likely to be the most well-known for its benefits on health. 100% pure extra virgin olive oil has been shown to improve beneficial cholesterol levels, reduce bad cholesterol, and improve heart health significantly. Olive oil is best used for stir-frying or low heat preparation since, under high heat, it may lose some of its natural health benefits.

Palm Oil

A relatively unknown type of cooking oil in many parts, it is extracted from the fruit of oil palm trees. Notably, red palm oil, in particular, is rich in Vitamin E and Coenzyme Q-10, potent antioxidants. The oil is very stable and is perfect for high heat cooking.

Avocado Oil

A rarely used oil with a high concentration of the antioxidant Vitamin E, it offers tons of benefits for both skin and heart. Extracted from the flesh of the avocado, as opposed to the seed like many other oils, the oil isrich in monounsaturated fats. These fats are perfect for the benefit of heart health. Avocado oil also contains another vital antioxidant, lutein, essential for maintaining the health of eyes. As if that's not enough, avocado oil is known to boost the absorption of fat-soluble vitamins, making it perfect for low carb diets.

Rice Bran Oil

Not often used in the West, but a traditional staple in Japan. This oil is very stable at room temperature and is also suitable for high-temperature cooking. Research has found that rice bran oil contains a unique antioxidant compound, which can help to improve cholesterol levels, in addition to its high content of unsaturated fats, which are the best for heart health. Keep in mind that rice bran oil is still calorie-heavy, so use sparingly. Generally, two to three tablespoons a day is advised.

Excluded Oils

You may have noticed the exclusion of two immensely popular oils, soybean, and canola. The reasons are simple; this is because these two oils are not considered good enough to be necessary for overall health. Most canola oils are highly processed "synthetic" versions of another oil and are produced using toxic chemicals.

Soybean oil, on the other hand, is too high in its omega-6 content, which is a fatty acid that promotes inflammation in the body, if it is not balanced out with Omega 3 Fatty Acids. Consuming too much Omega 6 can cause inflammation, hastening aging, disease, and many other undesirable conditions.

The Importance of Omega 3

There are many benefits of taking omega 3. The most beneficial one is it helps our mood swings, and It balances our hormones. Omega 3 Fatty Acids are crucial in maintaining a healthy inflammatory system.
Our body produces thousands of omega fatty acids, that is the benefit of taking them. When you want to improve your mood or the way you feel, take omega 3s and feel better.

Even though you need omega fatty acids for immune health to function at optimum levels, this is only part of the equation. If we start to feel off, or the situation we are in is not going well, then we will be more likely to overreact and have a negative mood. Also, many of us have experienced mood swings from extreme stress, which creates a release of stress hormones. These hormones are released into our bloodstream.

If these are not balanced, it could create a negative effect on our bodies. So, if the natural balance is damaged, then the body will react in a negative way. To improve your mood, you must get your body working properly by balancing the amount of omega 3 and other fatty acids in your blood. It also enhances your immune system to fight off infections and other problems that may arise.

By now, you will have heard a lot mentioned about leaky gut and the associated health problems it can cause. As a reminder, this is an autoimmune disease that attacks our body's defense system; it causes inflammation, and in turn, causes mood swings.

We are going to explain how eating foods that contain healthy fats and making sure we eat enough Omega 3 is essential to treating this autoimmune disease. We must take care of our bodies to maintain mood stability.

Leaky gut, of course, affects nearly all kinds of inflammatory diseases; it includes Multiple Sclerosis, Lupus, and Rheumatoid Arthritis. To treat these diseases, we need to get back our natural defense systems.
The fact is we are losing our body's ability to produce healthy fats and omega fatty acids because of the foods we eat. This becomes one of the largest causes of mood swings and irritability.

The best way to keep our bodies working properly and prevent these symptoms from arising is to help our body optimize its immune defenses with Omega 3 fish oil supplements. This will help keep the mind, body system working at its best.

Safe Foods, High in Omega 3 Fatty Acids

To get the best results with your Autoimmune Diet Protocol, you must understand the different foods that are high in Omega 3 fatty acids. There are foods that are naturally high in these acids, helping to prevent you from getting inflammation, allergies, and other conditions.

The first thing you need to know is that your body needs Omega 3 fatty acids in order to function with a healthy immune system. This nutrient is the most common and easily obtainable source of fatty acids and is present in many foods, such as:

- fish
- meats
- seeds
- nuts
- eggs
- avocados
- walnuts
- flaxseed
- and various kinds of fresh fruits and vegetables.

Speak with your doctor if needed, in order to make sure you are able to consume some of the foods on the above list, bearing in mind that this particular fatty acid is one of the most effective ways with which to absorb essential nutrients and vitamins.

A lot of researchers believe that having a higher consumption of food containing the correct nutritional value of fatty acids will help prevent the onset of many autoimmune diseases, including irritable bowel syndrome. This is because the immune system can more effectively fight off infection.

Some studies have also suggested that the Autoimmune Diet Protocol is beneficial in reducing the symptoms of arthritis. This is because the immune system is able to better identify and respond to the disease by sending out more appropriate signals to the joints.

Studies show that foods high in Omega 3 fatty acids, such as those mentioned on a diet, and including flaxseed oil and olive oil, can help to reduce the risk of developing inflammation in the joints. These foods have proven to provide pain relief and ease joint stiffness in people living with arthritis.
Olive oil, as shown earlier, offers an excellent form of Omega 3 fatty acids.

- Try a little olive oil drizzled over a salad.
- Are you cooking salmon? Drizzle a little olive oil across the top before popping it into the oven.
- Olive oil is an excellent natural anti-inflammatory agent that should not be overlooked due to its ability to assist the immune system.

Omega 3 Fatty Acids also help reduce free radicals in our bodies. Free radicals are one of the causes of inflammation and other diseases, and it is particularly good news that these nutrients help to protect against these agents.

The USDA (U.S. Department of Agriculture) has been considering the use of the DRI (Dietary Reference Intakes) as a standard for determining what a person should eat and how much to eat. This is the model used in a lot of research and has been helpful in making dietary recommendations.
You may be surprised to find out that a lot of vegetables have high levels of Omega 3 fatty acids,

which is surprising since we consider Omega 3's to come from food sources containing fats such as that found in fish.

- tomatoes
- carrots
- corn
- broccoli
- cauliflower. are just a few of the plant-based foods that have remarkably high levels of Omega 3 fatty acids.

These vegetables will add lots of vitamins and nutrients to your diet and also make your skin look bright, healthy, and well-nourished. Another bonus!

Chapter 6: Inflammation and our Moods

It may come as a surprise to some that sugar is being considered a major player in the inflammation of our bodies leading to disease and, in serious cases, disability. The reality is that the consumption of sugar is something that we choose to do through our meal choices, making it one of the easiest substances to eliminate. But also, the hardest.

If you sat up in bed tomorrow morning and declared out loud that you are no longer consuming candies; the hidden sugars in our diet in the form of condiments, and even so-called healthy salad dressings all remain hidden culprits in the war on sugar.

Even that glass of wine you enjoy on a Friday evening is not without sugar. In fact, the sweeter the wine, the higher the level of sugar. So, beware of those dessert wines. They are notoriously high in sugar content.
Artificial sweeteners are no help either, although they offer a reduced-calorie option, and they can certainly help in the reduction of calorie consumption, mainly if you are used to putting sugar in your iced or hot tea, and of course, your coffee, however many of the sugar substitutes contain the same chemical compound, chlorine, that is used in swimming pools. In those instances, as far as sugar is concerned between consuming chlorine,

or actual natural sugar, the choice would seem obvious. Chlorine, for most, would not be up for consideration!

For those of us managing an Autoimmune Disease, your health care professional will be able to advise you on your sugar intake in relation to the other foods you are able to eat, having established the foods you can eat via a process of elimination, or by following the Autoimmune Diet Protocol as described in this book.
However, for those of us who are searching for a more holistic path to overall wellness, to include a healthy, functioning immune system, it may be a more straightforward way of becoming mindful of the sugars we are eating and adjust accordingly from there.

In the pages of this book, there are several lists describing the kinds of food that help support a healthy immune system response.
Some of these foods contain natural sugars, which may, according to your dietary needs, provide a better alternative than sugar-laden treats.

- Did you know that if you freeze fresh grapes, they make a nice sweet treat? Great for a summer day and a better alternative than ice-cream!

Why is the Sugar to Mood Connection Important?

The problem is that even though we know that sugar affects our waistline, what we are only just really discovering is the connection between obesity and our immune system. Obesity can, as many know, lead to Type II Diabetes, placing further stress on our body. This additional stress involved with fighting associated side effects such as vision loss compromised nerve endings, and other related and often painful issues leave our body open to viruses and infection. In short, we run short of soldiers fighting the front lines.

As the chemicals in our body become disrupted, we become more addicted to the sugar present in our food. For those with Autoimmune Disease issues, this may lead to the Leaky Gut flare-ups we talked about in an earlier chapter; the mind-gut relationship becomes apparent as we start to feel depressed, low energy, and other mood compromising issues.

This may present to some as depression, with the predictable result of the issuing of anti-depressant and anti-anxiety medication prescription. To a nutritionist or a specialist medical professional looking at your diet, they understand the problem as related to the level of sugar consumed.

Of note, those who are dealing with obesity and Type II Diabetes issues, including sugar addiction, may benefit from a professional mental health provider who has experience and expertise in working with sugar-addicted clients. A chat with a health care provider will be able to provide the appropriate referral in these cases.

Sugar on the Brain

How does sugar affect the brain? Neurotransmitters are brain chemical messengers whose purpose is to carry messages from one neuron to another. Neurotransmitters perform a variety of functions in the body. These functions include the control of emotions, hunger, movement, and even the flow of blood to the heart.

Sugar has long been the source of many diseases. The American Heart Association, for example, has found that when blood sugar levels rise after a meal, many people experience depression. In fact, a number of studies show that those suffering from depression have significantly higher blood sugar levels after a meal than those not suffering from depression or symptoms of anxiety.

How does sugar affect the brain, and why does it affect some more than others? One theory suggests something to do with the Glycemic Index. This index measures how fast carbohydrates turn into sugar. This is particularly true of simple carbohydrates such as white pasta, rice, and bread whose starches turn into sugar much faster than the whole wheat variations of the above example.

It is believed that a low glycemic index may result in the release of neurotransmitters that are less likely to cause depression.

Essentially, the brain receives signals from the pituitary gland located in the back of the neck, and its function is to maintain the activity of the brain, particularly the secretion of neurotransmitters. When chemicals stimulate the brain, a signal is sent to the brain, requiring interpretation. This interpretation is then processed and released. For example, the brain releases hormones when the body experiences pain or emotion.

A second theory on how sugar affects the brain is called the glucocorticoid hypothesis. Glucocorticoids are natural chemicals produced by the adrenal glands in response to stress or physical injury. Because they prevent inflammation, they are also considered natural anti-depressants.

Glucocorticoids help the brain return to its normal state of function, therefore preventing depression. In support of this, there is a growing body of research indicating that people who regularly eat refined sugar have a heightened risk of depression. This is not to say all occurrences of depression are due to the presence of sugar in the diet. However, there is a growing body of evidence that supports a dietary link. Depression can also be caused by stress within the life of an individual.

However, when we consider the unhealthy food and sugar-laden alcohol choices we sometimes make when we are depressed or stressed out, sugar, may still make an appearance as a contributory culprit.

Avoiding Sugar to Boost your Mood

Insulin, a hormone that regulates sugar is spiked when we consume foods containing sugar. This is the case with cake or condiment; the result is the same. Insulin also makes our body crave sugar. Sugar consumption causes a temporary rush of insulin, which makes us feel full. The bad news is that this temporary rush of insulin puts us into a state of neuro inflammation, which is incredibly stressful on our immune system, resulting in some cases, an Autoimmune Disease.

Lactobacillus, a *good*-bacteria, helps maintain a healthy intestine. After consuming yogurt containing this substance, the helpful bacteria in the gut increases to the point where it can fight off against the buildup of harmful yeast in the body that can lead to a Leaky Gut. In doing so, it also neutralizes some of the unwanted effects of sugar.

Junk Food Kick Out!

Let us start with the obvious. Junk food is not suitable for our bodies. It is full of empty calories, so when we eat it, we cannot feel full, which means we eat more.
All junk food has one thing in common; it contains little to no nutritional value, resulting in our bodies not getting the nutrition it needs with predictable results.

One of the essential parts of a balanced diet is protein. When we consume junk food, our body is not getting the necessary nutrients required to build muscle or burn fat. When we consume enough

quality protein, it enables us to feel fuller for longer. Sugar, as we have seen, leads to spikes in our insulin and leads to hunger much faster than when we consume a quality meal.
Due to the number of empty calories in junk food, we add more weight to our body because we need to consume more of it to feel full.

A well-balanced diet, however, rich with protein and fiber, can make all the difference in not only our energy levels but our ability to sustain a healthy immune response.
So how can you stop eating junk food? With these simple tips.

- First, eat unprocessed, natural, whole food.
- Secondly, eat a variety of protein. Your body will take that as a sign that it is getting enough nutrients and will, therefore, be more inclined to burn the extra calories as fuel to keep you going.
- Snack on healthy seeds and nuts if you are not sensitive or allergic to these foods.
- Find sweet alternatives such as frozen blueberries and raspberries. Delicious on a hot day!

Chapter 7: Everyday Choices and Maintaining Good Nutrition for our Overall Immunity

It may come as a surprise to some reading this book there is a correlation between what we eat and how our immune system functions that the consumption of certain food does more than making us gain weight or affect our heart health. What we eat also can quite literally make us feel good or bad. Upbeat and full of energy, or moody and lackluster, as we have seen with the sugar connection.

In this chapter, we will take a deeper dive into our lifestyle choices, the food we take into our bodies and our immune systems.

Linking Poor Nutrition to Lowered Immune Systems

You may be wondering about the link between poor nutrition and lowered immune systems; in many cases, poor diet and reduced immune systems are inextricably linked.

In order to know the link between poor nutrition and lowered immune systems, you need to know how your body functions. We all know that the food we eat not only supplies us with essential nutrients but the nutrients are necessary for the correct functioning of the body.

There are nutrients needed for healthy tissue growth, so your cells are ready to make more enzymes and do what they have to do to produce energy for the rest of the body. In fact, there are many diseases caused by poor nutrition. These diseases include diabetes, heart conditions, various cancers, arthritis, and other immune diseases.

Poor nutrition weakens the immunity because our immune system is forced to function harder than it should.

Our immune system eliminates bacteria and viruses; this is important for keeping us healthy. When the system is compromised, through poor nutrition disease and illnesses take hold

Supplementing with vitamins, as we have seen, can be one way of sneaking essential vitamins into the body; however, that said, there can be no substitute for proper nutrition and the right foods for your wellness situation.

In addition to proper nutrition, we can also help our immune system through the elimination of harmful bacteria and the boosting of our good bacteria.

Several foods can help with this.

For example, you will eat yogurt rather than milk. This has been proven to be an excellent choice since the good bacteria in yogurt has shown to be greatly beneficial to the gut. Spicy foods can also help eliminate the harmful bacteria in the gut. Just make sure you can tolerate them.

Garlic, another excellent antibacterial agent, can also help boost the good bacteria, in addition to having other benefits such as maintaining proper blood pressure levels.

So, what foods should we eat in order for the maintenance of good bacteria in our gut? And the support of a healthy and responsive immune system?   The food list below may be able to help you with this.

As you read this list, bear in mind to think about the foods you can tolerate and focus on those. The list below assumes you are on the other side of the Autoimmune Diet Protocol, and you have, through the process of the controlled reintroduction explained in a previous chapter, established the immune-boosting foods you are able to tolerate comfortably.

Eat the Right Foods

Your diet is key to a healthy immune system. Fruits and vegetables provide Vitamins C and E, which help keep your immune system kicking along.

- Vitamin C is essential for white blood cells to destroy infection invading your body.

- Vitamin E keeps vital blood vessels working, enabling your body to transport blood to infected areas.

- Beta-carotene found in orange vegetables such as carrots, and other antioxidants are also found in fruits and vegetables. When your body processes food into energy, and even when you exercise, it creates harmful byproducts called free radicals. Over time, free radicals damage healthy cells in your body, causing disease. Antioxidants found in fruits and vegetables help neutralize free radicals keeping you healthy.

Vitamin C is often the first thing springing to mind when thinking about strengthening the immune system. During flu season each year, many of us hurry to the local pharmacy with the intent of purchasing some form of Vitamin C supplement.

Vitamin C, one of the most common and readily available supplements, comes in many forms, such as pills, powders, and even drinks. Like many other essential nutrients, Vitamin C can be readily supplied through a healthy diet alone, possibly making it one of the most accessible supplements to obtain.

A vast body of research supports the claim that Vitamin C is one of the most comprehensive vitamins one can take. Various studies have demonstrated that Vitamin C is not only great for the skin, in addition to acting as an aid in the prevention of infections, but it can also help resolve them once they are already present in the body!

Below is a list of foods rich in Vitamin C and in Vitamin E. Consume one or two portions of these daily and fill your immune-supporting daily quota!

Vitamin C Rich Foods

Many fruits and vegetables naturally contain high volumes of Vitamin C:

- Citrus fruit – oranges, lemons, limes
- Broccoli
- Cantaloupe
- Cauliflower
- Kiwi
- Papaya
- Red, green, or yellow pepper
- Sweet potatoes
- Strawberries
- Tomatoes
- Lychee
- Kakadu plums
- Acerola cherries
- Rose hips
- Chili peppers
- Guavas
- Blackcurrants
- Thyme

- Parsley
- Mustard spinach
- Kale

Vitamin E Rich Foods

- Sunflower Seeds
- Peanuts
- Oils: sunflowers, wheat germ, and olive oil
- Almonds
- Shrimp
- Hazelnuts
- Asparagus
- Broccoli
- Spinach
- Vegetable Oils

Antioxidant and Beta Carotene Rich Foods

- Dark leafy greens
- Kale
- Spinach
- Lettuce
- Carrots
- Sweet potatoes
- Broccoli
- Squash
- Cantaloupe
- Colorful peppers
- Apricots
- Peas

The Importance of Hydration

By now, you may have noticed how good habits can be beneficial regarding strengthening our immune system. Staying hydrated is another great example of how easy it can be to maintain our immunity and overall health.

Adequate hydration is paramount to fuel a healthy immune system. The mouth and throat being the first line of defense in the prevention of illnesses to include sore throats and other viral infections.

However, these body parts cannot optimally carryout their function in a state of dehydration. Furthermore, staying hydrated is essential to keep another integral part of the immune system working properly: the digestive system. Consuming enough fluids each day is vital to stay healthy.

Plant Rich Diets

Plant-based diets promote the wellbeing of our body by helping to detoxify, strengthen our immune system, and keep us from the damage of free radicals.

Free radicals are chemical molecules that attack the DNA within our cells. When the DNA is attacked, causing inflammation, the cells divide. This division leads to inflammation and, in some cases leading to diseases such as cancer, osteoporosis, heart disease, and even Alzheimer's disease. These free radicals attack and damage our cells by attaching themselves to the DNA, which leads to cell mutation.

Good diet and exercise are by far the best defense. However, the problem with exercise alone, in addition to some of the popular weight-loss diets is the lack of plant fiber that helps remove the free radicals the body produces.

- Plant rich diets are high in fiber, phytonutrients, antioxidants, vitamins, and minerals. The fiber in fruits and vegetables helps maintain healthy bowel functioning and the elimination of harmful waste material.

- The phytonutrients found in fruits and vegetables assist the body in the production of antioxidants. This helps fight off free radicals and, as we have seen, enhances our immune system. Antioxidants help prevent more damage to our cells, repairing DNA damage caused by free radicals.

- Protein is also important for the building and maintenance of our muscles. As we age, we lose the ability to maintain muscle mass, protein, along with exercise, can help maintain muscle mass as it is the building block of muscle tissue. Plant rich foods, because they are high in fiber, can help sustain a feeling of fullness for longer, thus making us more resistant to the temptation of snacking.

- For the best results when on a plant-rich diet, incorporate plenty of leafy greens and other plants into your diet. Always remember to drink water, and always include plenty of fruits and vegetables. These foods play an important role in creating a balanced diet, making a much healthier alternative to junk food.

Because of the benefits of a plant-rich diet, it is worth taking the time to plan your meals during the week. This will make you much more mindful of the food you are eating, and will also help prevent you from buying impulse junk food and quick meals that will do nothing to sustain you in the long term. Additionally, when we plan our meals and purchase the ingredients to make them, we become far more aware of how much sugar, and types of fats, and carbohydrates that we are pushing into our bodies. The health benefits alone over the long term are worth the effort.

In reality, it may not always be possible to do this. Life happens, even with the best of intentions; therefore, it may be helpful to at least aim for the eighty-twenty rule. In other words, eighty percent of the time, we consume the foods that are beneficial to our immune system. During the remaining twenty percent of the time, we may eat foods that may be less than ideal, but, have some nutritional value.

However, even then, it is essential to be mindful of individual tolerances for food and to remain true to that as much as possible to maintain a consistently healthy gut.

Obesity

A quick word about obesity: research has long pointed to obesity as being one of the key predictors of Type 2 Diabetes and its associated illnesses. What is also becoming clear is the link between obesity and inflammation, and ultimately the immune system. Inflammation can attack our organs and our joints, leaving us vulnerable to viral attacks because our white blood cells are busy fighting off the regular inflammation that is already present.

In other words, we are vulnerable to further attack from outside viruses and germs. Long term, a healthy diet will inevitably control weight, along with sensible exercise. The goal should always focus on healthy eating for a long time living.

Stress and our Immune System

When we do not have effective tactics to deal with stress in a healthy way, the body will react with the production of excess cortisol, an adrenal hormone associated with fight *or flight* responses.

The production of cortisol directly affects immune activity due to its production at the point of a stressful event. Cortisol also has evolved to allow our body to enter into a fasting mode during these times. The apparent lack of fasting today, leads to an increase in fat storage, along with a drastically lowered immunity.

There are herbal remedies designed to make us take it easy and relax. However, that is only part of the answer. The better solution is to become conscious of how we respond to stressful situations, improving our level of mindfulness at the same time.

Easier said than done, but becoming aware of what upsets us and how we are handling the stressful moment is key. Exercise can help, it gives a place for stress-induced adrenaline and cortisol to go, but a good supply of exercise-induced oxygenated blood to the brain can help with thinking ourselves toward a solution to a problem that might be bothering us.

Stress is going to be around us. However, being aware of what we allow ourselves to be pulled into, versus the things we can control can be a good beginning. If you know you are vulnerable to fast, negative responses, practice deep breathing exercises to allow for that exchange of blood rich oxygenated blood into the bloodstream. Slow, traditional yoga stretching can be great for this.

Take time for yourself even if it is a once per week spa bath or a quiet walk with the dog. Taking the time to take care of ourselves reminds us that we are valuable and can help calm the mind a little.

Taking the time to reward ourselves with a treat when we are going through stress can also be helpful. Again, the act of returning value to we can produce a flood of endorphins, also known as the *feel-good hormone.* Something simple is all that it takes; it does not have to be a mad spree at the mall! We do not want to add any problems you might be having!

Lastly, there are some people who, when they are stressed, become involved in community activities with a focus on helping others. Sometimes, the act of helping another can put things in perspective for us, helping us toward a solution for ourselves.

Other volunteer participants have expressed a sense of overall relaxation and wellbeing after working to help others. Why is all this important for our immune systems? Because the refocusing away from a negative, stressful response will reduce the level of immune compromising cortisol in our bodies.

Exercise for Immunity

When you develop and stick to an exercise routine, your health can improve far beyond any aesthetic appreciation you might receive! Your resting heart rate lowers to a healthier range, your digestive system pushes food through more efficiently, and it is more comfortable to sleep at night, making for a more revived you, in the morning!

Yet, there are plenty more effects that occur because of exercise that you might not even realize are taking place. And, the most important results are being discovered at the immune system level.

The Importance of Moving!

We might try to maintain a healthy lifestyle; unfortunately, there is not much we can do about the toxins in our physical environment and lurking within our food. When toxins build in our system, they can make us sick due to the suppression of our immune system's response.

For those of us with compromised immune systems, for example, anyone of the Autoimmune Diseases we have discussed, this can be a huge problem. Our body is already fighting against itself, to begin with, leaving little left to defend us against incoming viral bacteria from the outside world. Because of this, it is even more important to follow a healthy diet and a healthy lifestyle.

In some cases, Autoimmune Diseases such as Multiple Sclerosis and Rheumatoid Arthritis may make it difficult to follow traditional forms of exercise. This is fine; there are still exercises that you can do. The goal is to incentivize yourself to do them, even on days when mentally, you just do not feel like it.

A chat with your health care professional, and if appropriate, your physical therapist will be able to prescribe the right exercises for you. That may be yoga, which incorporates stretches and breathing within your range of ability. It may include water exercises such as aqua-aerobics or swimming, again according to your physical ability.

If walking is possible, then a thirty-minute walk or even a ten-minute walk per day will have far more benefits than remaining in the chair at home.   That said, if you are not able to move much beyond your chair due to physical restrictions or illness, simple chair stretches in place are far more beneficial then merely sitting and not moving our limbs at all.
The point is, is to do something as close to the ideal as possible, is better than doing nothing at all.

Sometimes the concentration involved in exercise is enough to make us feel better about ourselves even if we have not left the room. Just the ability to take time for ourselves can take our mind off the illness and can have huge benefits internally as far as our immune system is concerned. The endorphins that are produced through exercise are available to everybody regardless of the level of activity involved. In other words, you do not have to run a marathon to get positive results!

For those of us who are healthy, and are merely looking for an exercise to maintain overall health.

Then the best form of exercise is the one that we are going to stick with. For some, that may be a brisk walk with the dog after work, followed by a hike during the weekends. Somebody else may prefer to join the gym and take up a group exercise class during the week. Others may just enjoy running, followed by a yoga stretch on the return home. Others still, will prefer a more team-spirited sport, possibly rekindling a sporting activity that they used to do at school or college.

The bottom line is to do something.

Improving Blood Flow

When you exercise according to your level, your heart will work harder as your body starts to adapt to the exercise.

By improving your circulation or blood, you are allowing a much more considerable amount of blood to go through your veins in a shorter period. In the process, you are also forcing more of the healing, infection-fighting white blood cells to disperse throughout your body.

White blood cells, remember, are the body's first line of defense against infections or viruses. So, increasing the productivity and mobility of these white blood cells may assist with preventing infections or viruses that may already be brewing in your system.

Aging, Immunity and What We Can Do to Protect Our Overall Health

Our immune system needs to be in peak performance in order to protect our body from harmful bacteria and other nasty substances. These include various pathogenic toxins, bacteria, viruses, blood from another person, and even cancer cells.

The immune system is the part of the body that makes immune cells and antibodies that together destroy the harmful substances that can affect the body and cause disease.

Aging Affects the Function of Our Immune System

As we age, our immune system in all its complexities no longer works as well as they did during our younger years, unfortunately, like many things as we age. However, aging in an unhealthy way is not inevitable. There are changes or modifications that we can make now, that may have a positive effect in both the long and the short term.

- The immune system responds slower to the various antigens and pathogens exposed to it. This means we have a higher chance of becoming sick when exposed to a virus. In this case, things like flu shots may not work as well as expected or may only protect us for a short period of time. This is why the flu shot is often recommended to be given twice in the same season to elderly people, so the protection against the flu lasts longer.

- We may develop an autoimmune disorder. This is a condition of the immune system in which cells of the immune system make a mistake and attack the body's healthy tissues instead. As we have seen, there are many different autoimmune disorders, including Type I Diabetes, Rheumatoid Arthritis, Crohn's Disease, Grave's Disease, and Lupus.

- The body may not heal as fast. Our body contains fewer immune cells when compared to our younger days! Without an adequate number of immune cells, healing will be slower, resulting in an increased chance of a bacterial super infection from bacteria that get into lung tissue, for example. This could then lead to viral pneumonia.

- The body can lose the ability to detect and correct defects developing within the cells of the body. A cell is capable of mutating its DNA, for example, forming a cell that grows out of control to become a specific type of cancer. Older people are at a higher risk for cancer because their immune system fails to detect and recognize a cancerous cell. Once a cancerous cell develops, it allows the cell to

grow and divide into a cancerous growth or
tumor.

Prevention of Immune System Decline in an Aging Population

Despite all the doom and gloom, there are things we
can do to boost our immune system, even as we age.
These pro-active choices may help keep our immune
system strong so that it can help us heal better from
illness and prevent us from getting a disease in the
first place. Following are some things we might do to
boost the level of our immune system as we age:

- **Get the recommended vaccines.** In the
  elderly population, there are certain vaccines
  that are recommended, including the shingles
  vaccine, the pneumonia vaccine, and the flu
  shot, which is given annually and sometimes
  twice a year in the elderly. Your doctor will
  probably recommend these vaccinations to
  you. You may participate in these annual
  vaccinations if it is safe for you to do so.
  Consider these injections as future insurance
  against further immune damage.

- **Get plenty of aerobic exercise.** It has
  been determined that exercise can increase
  the effectiveness of the immune system. This
  means making sure you get approximately
  thirty minutes of aerobic exercise each day.
  Activities such as walking, running, or biking

during most days of the week will keep your muscles and heart strong and will boost the effectiveness of the immune system.

- **Eat foods that are healthy for you.** Correct nutrition is vital for a healthy immune system. Consuming a diet rich in vegetables, fruits, whole grains, and lean meats will help you get the protein and carbohydrates your immune system needs in order to protect your body against illness.
- **Stop smoking today.** Smoking cigarettes can compromise your immune system, making it weaker. When you smoke, you are especially more prone to getting lung infections.

- **Limit alcohol.** Alcohol can weaken the immune system; therefore, it may be a good idea to begin limiting the number of drinks you have to less than two alcoholic beverages per day so that your immune system can remain healthy.

- **Stay safe from falls and injuries.** Because your immune system is weaker, any time you are injured, you can expect to heal from these injuries more slowly than you would have if you were younger. Be careful during winter months when there may be snow and ice on roads and sidewalks.

It is no secret that maintaining a healthy immune system is critical to optimizing a good quality of life and overall well-being. This truth becomes even more apparent during times when there are pandemics and other immunity threatening diseases!

Most of the topics we discussed show a result in a strengthened immune system that is important for the health of the entire body. The positive correlation between general health and immune function is intricately linked on both sides of the equation.

- Anything harmful to your health is bad for your immune system.

- Likewise, any factor that is detrimental to your immune function is directly related to other health issues!

Below are habits we can implement today that will help ramp up our immune system and fortify our natural defenses against a wide variety of illnesses.

Get Good Sleep

We have all heard time and time again how important getting enough sleep is to our health. Besides not feeling terrible the next day, rest is responsible for a vast array of biological processes designed to heal and restore the body. One of these processes is related to your immune system. Sleep is especially essential for your immune system.

According to the European Journal of Physiology, sleep deprivation causes a stress response in the body that, among other issues, leads to chronic inflammation and significant immunodeficiency.

When we sleep, our body produces proteins called cytokines. Cytokines fight against infection, so getting enough sleep helps you maintain enough cytokines to fight germs.

Lack of sleep also decreases our immune system's overall function. Our body needs rest so we can use some of our energy to rebuild and strengthen the cells that fight disease. Getting enough sleep allows our body to share energy between active movement when we are awake and the rebuilding function of our cells and systems.

Outside of the research showing a direct link between lack of sleep and getting sick, we may have experienced this situation at some point in our own life. During particularly hectic periods in which we have been stressed and tired for days on end, we may come down with a viral illness, such as a cold or even the flu that only worsens our already stressful situation!

Managing Stress

Stress is a huge culprit to a compromised immunity, especially chronic stress. Choose from the stress management options below to help keep your stress levels down.

- Meditation
- Yoga
- Rest, relaxation, and leisure time
- Progressive muscle relaxation
- Guided imagery
- Tai chi/Qigong
- Deep breathing
- Practicing stillness of mind and body
- Engaging in activities you enjoy
- Movement and exercise

Protecting Ourselves Against Germs

Germs can be found not only in the air but on any surface around us. When someone who is sick coughs or sneezes, germs that are expelled may land on their hands or the area around them. If they touch things with their hands that have germs on them, they spread the germs around even farther.

Shared surfaces, like ATM keypads, gas pump handles, and door handles, can contain many germs. Germs cannot live forever on surfaces, but since germs are too small to see, we will never know they are there.

- Regular hand washing helps prevent any germs on our hands from entering our body through our mouth, nose, or eyes.

- Covering cuts and scrapes helps keep germs from entering open wounds.

- Washing vegetables and cooking meat to the proper temperature helps prevent you from ingesting germs too.

Why is this important to immunity? Because the presence of viruses in our systems can cause immune reactions that compromise our immune system, causing overactive reactions whereby our immune system turns in on itself. It is during these stressful moments on the immune system caused by viruses in the air that attack our bodies, particularly if we are run down through stress or through a pre-existing illness that further complications can arise, leading to further damage to both our organs and our immune system.

Practicing good hygiene, regardless of what is happening in the rest of the world, only makes sense if you stop and think about it. There is so much that we take for granted; we seldom take time to think about how our actions may be affecting our health in both the long and the short term. We think about what to eat, and we think about the right sort of exercise, and stress management techniques, however, we are not always as mindful as we should be about our day-to-day hygiene habits. When our immune system is compromised, daily hygiene habits such as basic hand washing hands after contact with surfaces, other people, touching our clothes and our hair becomes even more critical.

This does not mean that we become obsessive and compulsive, with respect to bacteria and germs. It is more out of regard for the devastation that a virus can produce within our system. It stands to reason that if we are going to take care of our immunity through our diet, that we should continue to extend a truly holistic approach and look at every aspect of our lives and manage where possible.

Conclusion

Thank you for reading *Autoimmune Protocol Diet*. I hope you have found it informative while at the same time, providing you with some practical tools that will help you both understand and implement the critical aspects of your Autoimmune Deficiency Diet Protocol.

Autoimmune diseases can affect anyone, sometimes triggered during times of extreme stress, or a simple virus that sends our immune systems into overdrive, causing our white blood cells to attack our healthy cells, leading to further inflammation and *flare-ups*.

Until recently, finding the right diet, was something of a hit and miss affair as most diets were focused primarily on controlling either fats or carbs to initiate weight loss. Beyond the so-called Mediterranean Diet, a diet focusing purely on reducing inflammation that can be beneficial for both medical and preventative reasons was, for many, a challenge to find.

In this book, I hope you have discovered some of the food and lifestyle answers you have been searching for, in addition to perhaps, inspiring you to be more mindful concerning lifestyle choices along with potential trigger foods, and even stress.

I am a great believer in passing good things along. So, if you would like to help someone like yourself, who is perhaps looking for answers, and help better to meet the requirements of their unique dietary needs.

We never know how much our words have the power to help someone else. To your absolute best health.

"Other books by Alexander Great"

Autoimmune Diet for Beginners*: Complete Step-By-Step Guide to Cooking Healthy Dishes and Losing Weight Quickly With the Autoimmune Diet:*
https://www.amazon.com/dp/B08D1VYW6F

Autoimmune Diet Cookbook*: Complete Step-By-Step Guide to Cooking Healthy Dishes and Increase Immune Defenses With The Autoimmune Solution:*
https://www.amazon.com/dp/B08D3Y66G7

Autoimmune Disease Anti-Inflammatory Diet*: 30 Healthy Anti-Inflammatory Recipes to Eat Well Every Day and Improve Health Fast Without Feeling on a Diet:*
https://www.amazon.com/dp/B08CYB3WWQ

AIP Diet : *4 Manuscripts: Autoimmune Protocol Diet, Autoimmune Disease Anti-Inflammatory Diet, Autoimmune Diet for Beginners, Autoimmune Diet Cookbook*
https://www.amazon.com/dp/B08JWP59MD

www.ingramcontent.com/pod-product-compliance
Lightning Source LLC
Chambersburg PA
CBHW070809240726
48654CB00007B/272